# *What's the fuss about ADHD?*

Dr Brendan Belsham

ISBN-13:
978-1479148899

ISBN-10:
147914889X

*To fellow parents*

# CONTENTS

# Introduction

Everyone has an opinion about it. If you mention the terms 'ADHD' or 'Ritalin' at a dinner party, you are bound to provoke lively debate. Try it. You would have much less fun with, say, diabetes and insulin, or asthma and inhalers. ADHD is a topic which evokes heated and varied opinion. It seems to be a convenient soapbox upon which many childhood and parenting issues are debated.

Attention Deficit Hyperactivity Disorder, to use its full title, refers to a condition in which a child (or adult) displays excessive inattentiveness, hyperactivity and impulsivity. These symptoms can occur in varying combinations, giving us three subtypes of the condition, namely the inattentive, the combined, and the hyperactive-impulsive subtypes. Studies suggest a worldwide prevalence of around six percent of school-going children. It seems to affect boys more than girls. We refer to the condition as ADHD, whether or not there is hyperactivity present. The term 'ADD' doesn't actually exist officially, although colloquially, it is often used to refer to children with the inattentive subtype of the condition.

But there is far more to it than that. When I first joined the ranks of child psychiatry, I saw ADHD as a 'grudge condition,' something I had to study but couldn't get excited about. I viewed it as dry and mundane, favouring the rarer, more exotic conditions, as many students do. But twelve years of private practice have changed my mind. At international meetings, it is not uncommon to be assailed by organised demonstrations voicing opposition to our conference, our 'pseudoscience' and our profession, which 'drugs children with mind-altering chemicals'. This initially shocked me, cacooned as I was within the cloistered confines of my university training. Clearly, these people did not sing from the same hymn sheet. Far from being dry and mundane, ADHD has increasingly become the touchstone for many issues in child psychiatry and for matters pertaining to children in general.

I am intrigued by this disconnect between the science of ADHD and the real world of public opinion. Surely the science speaks for itself? When working with parents – educated, intelligent people – I spend as much time unravelling rhetoric as I do addressing the condition. I find this both challenging and frustrating; challenging because such questions force me to sharpen my own understanding of the current research, and frustrating because a typical consultation doesn't allow me to do justice to a parent's need for proper information. This book is an attempt to meet this need by providing unbiased information about the condition, information which is neither 'dumbed down' at the one extreme, nor obscured by scientific jargon at the other.

In medicine, as in many other disciplines, technical terms interfere with the layperson's understanding; they are a barrier to access. Sometimes doctors even hide behind them, lest their own superficial grasp of concepts be exposed. But new words emerge and grow with the new discoveries in a field, adding to its richness and building the platform for future breakthroughs. Simply deleting them leaves us poorer in our understanding of important concepts. So in communicating science to the layperson, we need to carefully explain this jargon without losing the descriptive depth which it provides. To this end, I have been inspired by authors such as Malcolm Gladwell, Ben Goldacre and Bill Bryson; they are able to convey scientific findings in a manner which is both accessible and enjoyable.

It's not pseudoscience or rocket science, it's just science, and there's no reason why you should be denied access to it. The issues thrown up by ADHD and its treatment are important societal issues, and worth debating. So whomever you might be – a concerned parent, a fellow professional, or merely an interested observer – get on your soapbox, take up your megaphone, let's begin.

*Brendan Belsham*
*August 2012*

# 1

# Fidgety Philip and the history of ADHD

*... it is the disease of not listening, the malady of not marking, that I am troubled withal.*

Falstaff
King Henry IV, Part 2
Act I Scene II

Many parents ask me why ADHD was not around when they (or at least their grandparents) were at school. They are suspicious of a diagnosis which seems to be a recent fad, and alarmed at how many children are being prescribed medication for concentration difficulties. Indeed there have been accusations levelled at the pharmaceutical industry of having 'invented' the condition, after the fortuitous discovery of the cognitive benefits of the amphetamines. History does not support these claims, as we shall see.

## Once upon a time...

The concept of hyperactivity in children has been documented in the medical literature since the $18^{th}$ Century. In 1798, the Scottish-born physician and author, Sir Alexander Crichton, described what seems to be a mental state much like ADHD in his book *An inquiry into the nature and origin of mental derangement:*

*comprehending a concise system of the physiology and pathology of the human mind and a history of the passions and their effects* (which surely wins the prize for the most longwinded title in the history of academia). In this work, Crichton describes individuals with a 'disease of attention,' who refer to themselves as having 'the fidgets,' and have 'the incapacity of attending with a necessary degree of constancy to any one object,' hallmark symptoms of what we now call ADHD. He was also accurate in other aspects of his portrayal of the condition, such as its early onset and the possibility of improvement with maturity:

> *... it becomes evident at a very early period of life, and has a very bad effect...but it seldom is in so great a degree as totally to impede all instruction; and what is very fortunate, it is generally diminished with age.*

Furthermore, as the following excerpt reveals, he identified the tendency of such children to be easily bored with repetitive, unstimulating tasks, and how genuinely difficult it is for them, implying an innate rather than a willful lack of focus:

> *...it was obvious that they had a problem attending even how hard they did try. Every public teacher must have observed that there are many to whom the dryness and difficulties of the Latin and Greek grammars are so disgusting that neither the terrors of the rod, nor the indulgence of kind entreaty can cause them to give their attention to them.*

Alexander Crichton was a pioneer in the field, in fact about a hundred years ahead of his time in his observations. Where he was *really* ahead of his time, however, was the absence, in his writings, of any of the moralism introduced by later authors. He understood that these kids genuinely battled to concentrate despite their best endeavours. It would take 150 years for the scientific community to return to this viewpoint.

**Fidgety Philip**

In 1846 the German physician Heinrich Hoffman published a series of illustrated poems entitled *The Struwwelpeter*, variously translated as 'slovenly' or 'shock-headed' Peter. It is a series of morality tales, written for children, involving characters who get their respective comeuppances for various forms of bad behaviour. One of the protagonists, a boy named 'Fidgety Philip,' is described causing havoc at the dinner-table and generally exasperating his polite, over-dressed Victorian parents. Hoffman's descriptions and illustrations of young Philip and his household bear a striking resemblance to modern-day ADHD (except, of course, that modern families don't eat together anymore):

> *See the naughty restless child*
> *Growing still more rude and wild*
> *Till his chair falls over quite.*
> *Philip screams with all his might*
> *Catches at the cloth but then*
> *That makes matters worse again.*
> *Down upon the ground they fall*
> *Glasses, plates, knives, forks and all.*
> *How mamma did fret and frown*
> *When she saw them tumbling down!*

*And papa made such a face!*
*Philip is in sad disgrace.*

Note the use of judgemental terms such as 'naughty,' 'rude' and 'disgrace' which imply some sort of badness or moral failure. Such terms would never be seen in any modern description of ADHD, nor were they used by his predecessor Dr Crichton. The condition is now widely recognised as a neurobiological disorder rather than a character defect. One has to feel for poor Philip.

## The Goulstonian lectures

In 1902, the father of British paediatrics, Sir George Frederick Still, in his 'Goulstonian lectures,' described a group of children who would meet diagnostic criteria for modern-day ADHD. His findings were later published in the *Lancet*. These children had serious problems with sustained attention and self-regulation, showed little inhibitory volition, were excessively emotional or passionate and could not learn from the consequences of their actions, though their intellect was normal. Furthermore, he stressed their defiance and resistance to discipline, which he, like Hoffman, attributed to a moral problem:

> *I would point out that a notable feature in many of these cases of moral defect without general impairment of intellect is a quite abnormal incapacity for sustained attention... there is a defect of moral consciousness which cannot be accounted for by any fault of environment.*

Perhaps what he was getting at was the association between ADHD and what is now referred to as

4

Oppositional Defiant Disorder, or the more severe Conduct Disorder, a condition in which the child repeatedly violates the rights of others, often without remorse for his actions. Full-marks for that, George; as we now know, 40% of boys with ADHD have Oppositional Defiant Disorder, and around a third of these will develop Conduct disorder.

He was also correct in his observation that there is no obvious relationship between intelligence and ADHD symptoms. In fact, modern research *does* reveal an association between ADHD and lower IQ scores, but it only amounts to a few points and it is only evident when we study large groups of ADHD kids. At an everyday clinical level, ADHD is no respecter of intelligence quotient.

What Alexander Crichton originally termed a 'disease of attention,' and George Still a 'moral defect' has subsequently been known by a variety of other labels, including Minimal Brain Dysfunction (MBD), Hyperkinetic Reaction and Hyperkinetic Disorder (the British and Europeans still stubbornly refer to it as such). It was only as recently as 1987 that it received its current title Attention Deficit Hyperactivity Disorder. But the clinical descriptions of the condition have been remarkably consistent over the years. We are talking about the same entity.

**Arithmetic pills**

In 1937, Charles Bradley, a paediatrician working in Rhode Island USA, was treating children for headaches. He believed they were caused by a lack of spinal fluid (I can't imagine why), and prescribed benzedrine, an amphetamine, in an attempt to stimulate the production of this fluid. It was noted by the teachers and nurses who cared for the children that those who had received benzedrine showed an improvement in both behavior and academic performance. This was apparent even to the children, who began to call the medication 'arithmetic pills' as a result of the improvement in their studies. As with so many other medical breakthroughs, the discovery of the benefits of the amphetamines was an accident. (In case you were wondering, their headaches didn't improve.)

**A dodgy backhand**
But the wheels turned slowly, and it took a long time for this class of drugs to really catch on as a treatment for concentration and behaviour problems in children. In 1944 the chemist Leandro Panizzon, in the employ of the Swiss pharmaceutical company Ciba Geigy (now Novartis), synthesized the molecule methylphenidate in the laboratory. His wife Marguerite had low blood pressure and would take the drug as a stimulant before playing tennis, bless her. He named the substance Ritaline, after his wife's nickname, Rita. Sweet, isn't it?

Actually it wasn't his wife's backhand that inspired the development of the molecule, nor was it aimed at treating concentration, despite Bradley's earlier findings. It was in fact initially developed for use in chronic fatigue, mild depressive states, and narcolepsy, a condition in which the sufferer falls asleep at inappropriate times. So in 1954 Ciba Geigy registered Ritalin for use in adults with these conditions.

It was only in 1963, however, that methylphenidate was first marketed for children, in the form of 'Ritonic,' a curious mixture of methylphenidate, vitamins and hormones. In the same year, the results of the first properly conducted trials of Ritalin (pure methylphenidate) for what was then called 'hyperkinetic reaction' were published. The results were unequivocal; Ciba had a winner. And so, over a century and a half after the first clinical descriptions of the condition, Ritalin came into widespread use for the treatment of concentration problems in children.

And the rest, as they say, is history.

# 2

# 'Please test him for ADHD'

The teacher reports that your child is underachieving in the classroom, and suggests an assessment. It may have been a series of phonecalls, possibly from several teachers over the years, and you are feeling increasingly hounded. Over time, you start to fear any contact from the school, knowing what it's likely to be about.

Like any parent, you are likely to respond emotionally. After all, we don't enjoy receiving criticism about our children, however well-intentioned. It is natural to go on the defensive, and parents often begin by blaming either the teacher or the school. Sometimes feedback about our children awakens issues which we experienced ourselves years ago in the classroom; our reactions are emotional and irrational because they have been amplified by such (often subconscious) memories.

As a practitioner, I have often found myself caught in the middle between a teacher's concerns and a parent's denial. Indeed, many families come to see me under duress, having been issued a thinly-veiled ultimatum to have their child assessed, 'or else!' This is a far from ideal beginning to a doctor-patient relationship, and I often have to spend a large chunk of the first consultation rescuing this tense situation.

But it doesn't have to be this way. How the teacher approaches you as a parent can facilitate the process. There is a world of difference between 'I think Johnny should go onto Ritalin' and 'I have noticed that Johnny often daydreams in class and doesn't finish his work. How about we ask a specialist to look into this?' I know which I would prefer.

### Who does the diagnosing?

Parents are often unsure about this, as there are at least three different medical specialists to whom you might be referred. Schools often refer to these specialists somewhat interchangeably and randomly, further compounding parents' confusion. The truth is, any of the following doctors would be appropriate:

1.  A child and adolescent psychiatrist; that is a psychiatrist who has specialised in children's conditions;
2.  A neurodevelopmental paediatrician; that is a paediatrician with a special interest in ADHD; or
3.  A paediatric neurologist; that is a neurologist with expertise in childhood neurology.

For completeness, one should probably also include the general paediatrician and family doctor (GP), although you must do your homework because not all generalists have expertise with this condition. But in our context of scarce resources (at least in South Africa), it is only pragmatic that some of the load should be shared by our colleagues.

Many parents are referred specifically to a neurologist because the teacher feels they need to have an EEG (an electroencephalogram), a procedure which records the electrical activity of the brain. Now, please concentrate because I am only going to state this once:

*You cannot diagnose ADHD with an EEG.*

Anyone who tells you otherwise is either deluded or practicing quackery. There is certainly a place for the EEG, for example if it is suspected that the child has absence or petit mal seizures, a type of epilepsy in which the brain 'switches off' for short periods of time. In such instances the EEG is an appropriate diagnostic test. But please don't let anyone tell you that your child has to have an EEG, including the latest fad, the quantitative EEG (known as the 'qEEG'), in order to diagnose ADHD.

There is something vaguely unsatisfactory about not having a 'sciency' test to diagnose a condition – which no doubt contributes to the proliferation of gimmicks such as the qEEG – but unfortunately that is where we stand. The diagnosis involves a checklist of symptoms which should be evident in the child *and* which should be causing significant impairment in his or her daily functioning. The latter clause is particularly important as it guards us against over-diagnosing the condition – we call this 'false positives' – or worse, degenerating into cosmetic pharmacology, the perils of which we return to in a later chapter.

**The DSM IV**

Now, without further ado, allow me to introduce you to the Diagnostic and Statistical Manual of Mental Disorders, better known as DSMIV (it is now in its fourth edition). Published by the American Psychiatric Association, this is the 'bible' of psychiatric disorders. The other major classification system, used mainly in the UK and Europe, is the International Classification of Diseases (now in its 10th Edition, hence ICD10). We will restrict ourselves to the DSMIV, as the more widely used of the two. This tome records the diagnostic rules for any condition you care to mention. In the section describing childhood conditions, you will find that the symptoms of ADHD are divided into three clusters. Here are the nine symptoms of the inattentive cluster:

1. *An abnormally short concentration span;*
2. *A frequent resistance to sustained mental effort, especially with boring or repetitive tasks;*
3. *Easy distractibility;*
4. *Marked forgetfulness;*
5. *A tendency to lose things frequently;*
6. *Difficulty organising tasks and poor planning;*
7. *Not listening properly to instructions;*
8. *A tendency to rush work, giving poor attention to detail and making frequent careless mistakes;*
9. *Often not completing tasks*

**'But there is nothing wrong with his concentration in front of the TV'**

Most of these symptoms are self-explanatory, but this particular objection is so common that I must address it. It is true that a child with ADHD may concentrate very well in certain situations, even *too well* at times. It is known that such children often 'hyperfocus' on certain tasks, to the exclusion of other, more important or relevant activities. The problem is thus not necessarily an absolute inability to concentrate, as it is an avoidance of boring or unstimulating tasks, which differ from the child's agenda! This has to do with the executive system of the brain, which governs higher functions such as prioritizing, delay of gratification and time management. We will encounter it again in chapter four.

In its wisdom, DSMIV has decreed that a child should display at least six of these nine symptoms to warrant the diagnosis. There is nothing magical in this particular threshold, and good studies have shown that children with only four or five symptoms may be as impaired as children with seven or eight criteria. So this cut-off is quite arbitrary, and on another planet it might be four or eight. But we have to have some sort of guideline, so six it is.

And here are the criteria for the other two clusters:

**Hyperactivity**
1) *Constantly on the go, "as if driven by a motor"*
2) *Runs about or climbs excessively*
3) *Restless, unable to stay seated*
4) *Fidgets excessively*
5) *Excessively talkative*
6) *Plays loudly*

**Impulsivity**
7) *Often interrupts or intrudes on others*
8) *Cannot wait his or her turn*
9) *Blurts out answers before the question is completed*

Again, the powers that be have decided that six of these nine symptoms are sufficient to diagnose the hyperactive-impulsive subtype of the condition, or, together with six of the inattentive symptoms, the combined subtype.

In assessing these criteria, the doctor should

directly observe the child in the consulting room, usually involving some form of structured activity, such as drawing or writing. It is also very important to interview the child directly. Children are notoriously poor at judging their own concentration, so we can't rely exclusively on this feedback, but they do give us other important information, such as their experience of school and the quality of friendships and family interactions, which are important aspects of the subjective distress and impairment due to the condition.

## Safety in numbers

The decision as to whether or not a child 'qualifies' for a given symptom is essentially a subjective one. This is why it is so important to receive as much feedback as possible from the various adults involved in the child's life. If the teacher, the doctor, both parents and the soccer coach all feel that the child is unusually distractible for a seven-year-old, then one can be confident enough to tick that box. But if only the teacher notices this symptom, at odds with everyone else, then one should be far more cautious.

## Rating scales

To this end, we tend to use rating scales to assist us in making the diagnosis and monitoring progress. Standardised questionnaires are commonly used for this purpose. There are several to choose from; I use the Conners or the Copeland rating scales. They are tabulated checklists of symptoms, asking for the degree to which the child displays each symptom. But I must stress that questionnaires alone cannot make the diagnosis; they are tools to be supplemented with clinical judgement.

**A dimensional condition**

As you will no doubt have noticed, the symptoms listed above are displayed by *all* children from time to time, especially more immature children. Furthermore, in developmental conditions such as ADHD, the degree to which a trait is perceived as abnormal is influenced by the developmental stage of the child. Take impulsivity for example. I expect my four-year-old son to have a lower frustration tolerance than his ten-year-old brother, and to lash out from time to time. It is appropriate for his developmental stage. This symptom needs to be *really* severe, and out of keeping with his peers at preschool, for it to 'count' as an ADHD symptom.

It is also very important to stress that ADHD is a *dimensional* condition. Unlike other disorders in medicine, there are no clear-cut, neatly defined boundaries between illness and health. Rather, the symptoms we see in this condition occur in the population on a spectrum, with a so-called *zone of ambiguity* in between clear-cut cases and those who are obviously not affected.

This is in contrast to *categorical* diagnoses, such as haemophilia, for example. You can't have a 'touch' of haemophilia; you either have it or you don't. Likewise meningitis; you're either in or you're out. ADHD is not like that, and indeed, much of psychiatry is not like that. At either extreme of the spectrum the diagnosis is easy; it is relatively straightforward to diagnose the most hyperactive child and to confidently refute the diagnosis at the other end of the spectrum. But in the middle - around the zone of ambiguity - it is usually much more difficult.

**Temperament**

What we are grappling with here, essentially, is the dividing line between normal and abnormal. And this is where we must also consider temperament. As opposed to personality, which emerges over time, temperament refers to those traits and behaviours which appear in the first year of life. Several decades ago, child psychiatrists Stella Chess and Alexander Thomas identified nine distinct dimensions of temperament, which all exist on a spectrum in each individual. Here they are:

1. *Mood*
2. *First reactions (approach or withdrawal)*
3. *Adaptability (flexible or rigid)*
4. *Intensity (excessive or muted response to situations)*
5. *Rhythmicity or regularity*
6. *Frustration reaction (easily frustrated or persistent)*
7. *Sensitivity*
8. *Activity level*
9. *Distractibility*

I'm sure you noticed that several of these dimensions overlap with ADHD symptoms. Yet temperament is normal and ADHD is abnormal. What's going on here?

**Functional impairment**
These aspects of ADHD – the overlap with temperament and immaturity, the dimensional nature of the condition and the lack of an objective measurement tool – together mean that we have to pay very close attention to the concept of functional impairment. If we are to justify the inclusion of ADHD as a psychiatric disorder, there has to be, well, disorder!

There remains a vociferous minority who accuse the medical fraternity of something called *reification*, which means falsely calling something an entity which isn't actually a real entity. They say we have invented it for sinister purposes, arbitrarily lumping a group of symptoms together. I won't waste too many words on this, but if you need a rebuttal, you don't have to look further than the very obvious suffering associated with ADHD. A hallmark feature of any proper medical condition is that it is associated with distress and impairment in daily functioning, and ADHD has this in abundance.

Broadly speaking, there are three important domains of functioning to think about. We will start with academic performance. ADHD causes children to underperform in the classroom. This is especially important in the early grades, when foundational skills are being learnt. If ignored for too long, the resultant gaps in the child's learning can be very difficult to address later on. ADHD can affect the brightest children, the slowest, and anyone in between. But whatever the child's intelligence, it will cause them to underachieve relative to their potential.

Some bright children with ADHD seem to cope well enough in primary school when there is enough support in place, from both teachers and parents. If they are not particularly hyperactive, the teacher will not have had any reason to recommend an assessment. These children may only start to struggle in high school, when they are expected to be more organized and to work more independently.

Secondly, this condition often affects the social functioning of the child. This is usually the result of hyperactivity and impulsiveness, affecting how he interacts with his friends, his siblings and authority figures. He often alienates himself from his peers and may be genuinely unaware of why this has happened. Many children with ADHD are particularly defiant, and as mentioned in the previous chapter, a significant percentage of them have co-existing Oppositional Defiant Disorder. But even children who are purely inattentive have social difficulties; as you can imagine, their poor concentration affects their ability to track conversations and follow the rules of games, in effect sidelining them from their classmates' activities.

And thirdly, as a consequence of the above, these children are often distressed and demoralized. Their absentmindedness often gets them into trouble with parents and teachers alike. Their academic difficulties frustrate everyone including themselves, and they struggle with rejection from peers. Many can become clinically depressed, further compounding their problems.

If an inattentive or hyperactive child is not impaired in any of these areas then it is preferable not to make the diagnosis. After all, we can't go around diagnosing every absent-minded child with ADHD, now can we?

# 3

# Orchids and dandelions

With eighteen possible symptoms in various combinations, and functional impairment in several possible settings, it should not surprise us that ADHD is not a 'one size fits all' diagnosis. It presents in many different ways. As befits any such multifaceted condition, ADHD has a number of contributing causes and risk factors, operating in various combinations depending on individual circumstances. Nature and nurture both seem to be involved.

## The heritability of ADHD

The accepted dogma is that ADHD is a genetic condition, that it is inherited from one or both parents. But a closer look at the research reveals much more than this trite statement conveys.

The family study provides our first line of evidence. Close relatives (immediate family) of an ADHD child have been found to have an approximately five times increased risk of having it themselves. But sceptics were quick to point out that this clustering of ADHD within families could be due to shared factors in the home environment, so what was needed was a way of controlling for these environmental factors. Twin studies provide the means to do this, to tease apart the relative contributions of nature and nurture. Identical twins share

100% of their genes, and non-identical twins fifty percent. If the identical twin-pairs show more similarity in their symptoms than the non-identical twins, it follows that there is a genetic component at play. And many twin studies have in fact shown this to be the case. Adoption studies have provided us with further evidence. If the environment was the only causative factor, one would expect adoptive children (especially those adopted at birth) to be more like their adoptive families. But numerous adoptive studies show that adopted children are more similar to their biological relatives than to their adoptive relatives, on various measures of ADHD.

**Neuroscience 101**

Having established the heritability of ADHD, researchers began to focus on which particular genes are to blame. But before we get there, we need to digress and learn something about genes and about how the brain works.

A gene is the basic unit of heredity and is the vehicle for transmission from one generation to the next. Each gene comprises a sequence of DNA (a highly specialised chemical sequence) which codes for a particular protein, which in turn has some functional role within the cell and organism. We all have many genes (about 30,000), inherited from our parents, coding for the many characteristics or traits which make us unique individuals. In every cell, there are two copies of each gene, one from the father and one from the mother.

For our purposes, we will focus on those genes which play a role in brain functioning, and more specifically, in areas of the brain which are known to be affected in ADHD. And those brain regions are primarily the cerebellum and prefrontal cortex. (The term 'cortex' refers to the superficial layer of brain cells, as opposed to the deeper structures below.)

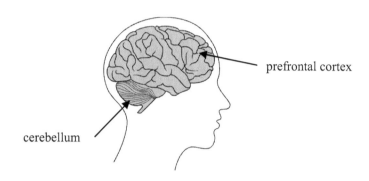

prefrontal cortex

cerebellum

**Figure 1**

These areas of the brain (figure 1) have been implicated in ADHD by means of sophisticated imaging studies (MRI scans and the like), which are able to sensitively measure the volume of the brain and its components.

Now, let's imagine we're looking at a piece of brain under the microscope. What you would see is lots of individual cells (in the brain we call them *neurons*), communicating with each other across minute gaps called *synapses*.

Direction of transmission

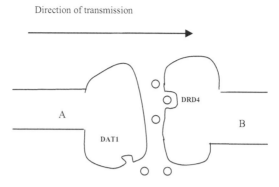

**Figure 2**

Figure 2 shows (highly schematically) two such neurons (A and B) with a synaptic space in between them. Numerous such communicating neurons contribute to pathways, or circuits, which allow for different areas of the brain to 'talk' to each other. There are a myriad of chemical messengers (called neurotransmitters) in the brain, which facilitate this communication between neurons. These include serotonin, noradrenaline and dopamine, to name but a few. Dopamine and to a lesser extent noradrenaline seem to be the most important in ADHD. In figure 2, the little circles are the neurotransmitters. Let's pretend they represent dopamine.

After having been produced in neuron A, dopamine exits the cell membrane, works its way across the synapse and communicates with neuron B. It does so by attaching itself to a dopamine receptor protein on that neuron. There are several dopamine receptors; I have chosen DRD4 (dopamine receptor D4). Dopamine 'docks' on the receptor, which in turn triggers a series of events in neuron B, allowing the communication to continue along the circuit. In this manner, the message is transmitted from one area of the brain, along a pathway, to another area.

The amount of dopamine in the synapse – and hence available to communicate with neuron B – is closely controlled by a very neat feedback system. Excess dopamine is 'mopped up' by another receptor on neuron A, which allows the reuptake of dopamine back into itself. In our example, it is called the dopamine transporter protein, DAT1 for short. This protein plays a starring role in ADHD treatment, providing the site of action of the stimulant medications.

**Hunting for culprit genes**
But now, back to the matter at hand. Because all cells in the body carry the full complement of genetic material, it is possible to take a sample of blood or other tissue from an individual and through clever technology, ascertain which genes you have or don't have. But of all the 30,000 genes to consider, where to start?

As luck would have it, researchers were handed an important clue, in the form of methylphenidate, better-known as Ritalin. We know two important things about this drug; one, that it is effective in treating ADHD symptoms (calm yourself, we'll discuss it later), and two, that it affects dopamine levels in the synapses between brain cells. So it was only logical to start looking at genes involved with dopamine, and... Voila! Enter the dopamine receptor gene, the gene which codes for the dopamine receptor protein, DRD4.

## The 7-repeat variant

As with any gene, we all have two DRD4 copies, one from each parent. These parental copies of genes are referred to as 'alleles' (pronounced al-*eel*). Thus for each gene, you will have two alleles. These alleles often differ, emanating as they do from two different people, and hence two different gene pools. One of the variants of the DRD4 gene is known as the 7-repeat allelic variant, so named because of a specific pattern observed in the DNA sequence. We will call it 7R for short.

If you take a group of kids with ADHD and compare them to a group of unaffected children, significantly more of those with the condition will have this offending, 7R allelic variant of the DRD4 gene. Now, not every child with ADHD has this allele, and not all with the allele have ADHD. But generally, children and adults with this genetic variant tend to be more novelty-seeking, impulsive, restless and inattentive than those without it.

Other genes have also been implicated in ADHD, including the gene coding for the dopamine transporter, DAT1. Because there are several genes involved in ADHD, it is referred to as a polygenic disorder, as opposed to certain other conditions, such as cystic fibrosis, for example, which is caused by one specific genetic variant.

## But it's not all about genes

Overall, twin and adoption studies reveal a genetic contribution of 70-80% to the observed symptoms of ADHD, which means that a significant chunk must be non-genetic, due to environmental factors. Several such environmental factors have been identified, and they all seem to operate really early on in life.

As early as the womb. A mother's smoking in pregnancy, for example, is a strong independent risk factor for her offspring having ADHD, even when you control for genes and other environmental factors. Other risks in pregnancy include alcohol consumption and maternal stress. Prematurity and birth complications, resulting in insufficient blood flow and oxygen to the brain, are additional risk factors for ADHD, even when there is no obvious brain damage in the aftermath of the delivery.

Other medical causes include epilepsy, brain infections including encephalitis, HIV/AIDS and various congenital and genetic conditions.

**The plastic brain**
In the first two years of a child's life, vital neurobiological changes are occurring. The infant's brain is highly 'plastic,' which means that it is changing and remodelling constantly. It is also growing at a fast rate; by the age of two, the brain is already 80% of its adult size. This is also the period when neuronal pathways receive a thick outer covering called *myelin*, which allows for faster and more efficient transmission of impulses. By the age of fifteen months, the density of synapses in certain areas of the brain (such as, you guessed it, the prefrontal cortex) reaches its peak, after which growth slows down. Thereafter, there is more refinement, reorganisation and 'pruning,' a process by which – as in the garden – inefficient neurons and synapses are culled.

Meanwhile, in parallel with these biological brain events, the crucial process of attachment is unfolding. Some famous simians will set the scene for us.

## Harlow's monkeys

Not too long ago – at least in Victorian times – the accepted approach to parenting a newborn child was to pretty much steer clear of it. Well, not quite, but there was a strong school of thought which warned that too much physical contact and comfort would spoil the child and interfere with the process of becoming independent. Any perceived bonding with the mother was solely due to her role as the food provider.

Thankfully, Harry Harlow and his classic experiments with Rhesus monkeys in the 1950's, helped to revise this coldly Pavlovian view of childrearing. He took infant monkeys and separated them from their mothers. When frightened, these infants had two available options, a wire-mesh surrogate mother which provided meals on demand, or a furry terry cloth surrogate, without food. They overwhelmingly chose the latter. This seminal work helped lay the foundation for attachment theory, a neglected area in child psychiatry, and I dare say, in parenting generally.

## Attachment

Attachment refers to the close emotional bonds of affection which develop between babies and their primary caregivers. In contrast to bonding, which is one-way, from mother to baby, and can be instantaneous, attachment refers to what happens in the child, and develops over a period of time. A newborn baby can be handed to anyone with no distress, but over the next few months the baby begins to show a preference for, and seeks out, a specific person. This is the beginning of attachment. Children will form attachments to various people over time, but the first and most important attachment relationship is almost always with the mother.

25

There are critical periods – a timetable, if you like – during which aspects of attachment should be occurring. By about 18 months, the attachment experience is then 'wired in,' and the consequences are far-reaching. There seems to be a biological programming effect of early experiences, which links these physiological and psychological processes. When we discuss the Romanian adoptees in the next chapter, we will encounter some compelling evidence to support this contention.

## Becoming securely attached

Depending on what happens between the mother and child in these crucial early months, children may become either securely or insecurely attached. If the mother is erratic, unpredictable, or unavailable, healthy attachment cannot occur. This is why it is so important to recognise and treat postnatal depression, a condition in which the mother cannot provide the emotional availability which her child requires.

To become securely attached, an infant requires a primary caregiver who is consistently present, and attuned enough to the child to respond appropriately to her needs for focused attention, physical affection and stimulation. Healthy attachment leaves the child with an 'internal working model,' or template, which allows her to see herself as valued, and others as 'basically good.' This facilitates healthy relationships in childhood and later life. It is a built-in protection against many social pitfalls, including bullying.

In addition, studies have shown that securely attached children have longer attention spans and show more persistence in tasks. Interesting findings, considering that children with ADHD show impairments in these very areas. There is actually very little in the scientific literature on this, but the few studies which have been published, support an association between insecure attachment and ADHD.

## Healthy attachment doesn't require a PhD
Please don't despair! Being a new parent is fun and if you just relax and enjoy your child, much of the above will happen spontaneously. One of the leading theorists in the field, Donald Winnicott, put it so well when he coined the term, 'The Good Enough Mother,' meaning that you don't have to be an expert, you just have to be, well, good enough. Perhaps your child didn't have the most optimal early months. Parenting is far more than attachment, and there are well-documented strategies which can influence your child for good even after the attachment phase. Read on!

## Expressed emotion
Another vitally important aspect of the child's psychological environment is the emotional milieu of the home. I find the term 'expressed emotion' confusing and unhelpful, but it does describe an important concept, so we had better stick with it. In essence, it refers to an observational measure of the emotional relationship between two people. The way parents talk about their children is indicative of how they interact with them, and can be quite accurately measured using a speech sample. In practice, I have found this to be true. In fact, it can often be ascertained in a consultation by a parent's opening statement, such as 'I'm going to kill him!' (just to clarify, that counts as bad!).

Apart from maternal hostility, other aspects of a relationship characterised as 'high expressed emotion,' (a clumsy term, don't you think?) include high levels of criticism and a lack of maternal warmth. Whilst this has not been identified as a causative factor in ADHD, it certainly affects the prognosis, mediating the progression to more serious behavioural disturbances such as conduct disorder. The converse is also true; maternal warmth in particular, seems to predict a better outcome in kids with ADHD.

### Finding middle ground

So, the available evidence suggests that both nature and nurture are important. Broadly speaking, psychiatrists and neuroscientists plug the former, and psychologists the latter. For the past fifteen years or so, the prevailing theory linking these competing theories has been the so-called 'stress-diathesis model.' You may have inherited the bad gene, say the 7R allele of the DRD4 gene, but this doesn't doom you. Only if circumstances turn sour will the gene be triggered, resulting in the unwanted condition. This implies an *interaction* between the environment and the genome, and indeed there has been a slew of research confirming this interaction over the past decade, in ADHD and several other psychiatric conditions.

### The Edison Gene

But it gets more interesting. There are some dissident views out there. An intriguing aspect of this 7R allele is that it is so common. And it *is* common, one study estimating the prevalence to be around fifteen percent of the American population. As Charles Darwin taught us, any genetic variant which confers a disadvantage on the individual and species should be selected out over time and become exceedingly rare, perhaps confined to isolated populations. Why hasn't this happened? According to Thom Hartmann, author of *The Edison Gene*, DRD4 kids (as he affectionately calls them) are actually essentially normal, but are forced to operate in a society which eschews the very qualities which hyperactive kids bring to the table: novelty-seeking, restlessness, risk-taking and the like. Qualities better suited to an age when we were hunters rather than sedate, risk-averse office workers who pay their taxes on time and whose children sit quietly in classrooms and listen to the teacher. He cites several examples of individuals who have done great exploits, who would meet modern day criteria for ADHD, Thomas Edison being one of them. Hartmann argues that these very traits which annoy primary school teachers are the traits needed to challenge the status quo and pioneer societal advances. They just need to be nurtured.

**Orchids and dandelions**
Support for Hartmann's view comes from a relatively new theory of genetics, called the orchid hypothesis (also known as the plasticity hypothesis), lucidly summarised by David Dobbs in an article entitled *The Science of Success*. The concept of 'dandelion children' has been around for a while, describing kids who are resilient and will cope in most circumstances. They won't shoot the lights out, but they will be okay even with average care. In contrast, 'orchid children' are particularly sensitive to their rearing conditions. Given the right environment, they bloom spectacularly, but if neglected they quickly wither and wilt. Whether good or bad, the environment has a pronounced effect on how they turn out.

Every society needs a healthy mix of both. Orchid kids have the high risk alleles such as 7R DRD4, and hence are more at risk for conditions such as ADHD. But these same risky genes carry with them a potential upside, which comes to the fore at certain crisis moments in the life of the individual or society. Provided they have been well-nurtured, that is. And there is good evidence to back this up, from several studies. Compared to children without the DRD4 7R allele, the behavior of those with this variant has been found to be more sensitive to the quality of parenting received, and to have a better treatment response to parenting interventions.

The orchid hypothesis might explain the high frequency of such alleles in the general population, answering Hartmann's objection and providing a neat reconciliation with the principles of natural selection. These risk alleles confer a sensitivity, not only to negative experience, as the stress-diathesis model would have it, but to *all* experience. They open the window wider, not just to the adverse environment, but to the whole environment, good or bad. This is both scary and exciting. The stakes are high, and getting the environment right just became a whole lot more important, at least for a certain group of kids. I hope you are getting the sense of how interrelated are the environment and the genome. And we are about to take it one step further.

**Genetic volume control**

In recent years, geneticists have discovered an increasing number of environmental influences which can actually *change* gene activity. Furthermore, these changes – known as epigenetic changes – can be transmitted from one generation to the next. Both the physical and the psychological environment can have such effects. There are a number of mechanisms by which these gene changes can occur. One example is *methylation*. A methyl group is a basic unit in organic chemistry: one carbon atom attached to three hydrogen atoms. It takes only the addition of a methyl group to a specific spot on a gene, to tell it to switch on or off, to shout loudly or to whisper.

Until now, we have all thought in a somewhat fatalistic and deterministic manner about our genetic makeup; that it's the hand we've been dealt and we just need to suck it up and move on. Not so, it seems. What this means is that the choices we make can influence the expression of our genes for better or worse, having an influence on the generations to come. I hope you are as excited about that as I am.

It works something like this. You inherit a particular gene from one of your parents, let's say the 7R DRD4 variant. It turns out that the expression of that gene is not a given. Rather, there are several environmental factors which might determine how influential it becomes. For example, if mom is extremely stressed in the pregnancy, her stress hormones, including cortisol, cross the placenta, enter your bloodstream and then your developing brain. These unusually high levels of cortisol cause your 7R gene to get methylated, thus activating it, and manifesting down the line with the clinical condition of ADHD. Your younger brother inherits the exact same allele, but by then the financial problems and dad's alcohol abuse have been sorted out, and a tranquil pregnancy ensures that his 7R variant remains quietly in the background.

### 'It's the environment stupid!'

I didn't say that. An eminent neurobiologist did, in one of his editorials. But I agree with him. For all the genetic vulnerability, it's the environment that has the final say, through its influences on brain development and gene expression. So much so, in fact, that 'nurture' can take a 'risk' allele like 7R DRD4, and actually turn it around for good, as in the orchid hypothesis.

So the next time you discuss this at a dinner party

you are entitled to say that the 'nature versus nurture' debate is actually so last century. The answer lies in a complex set of interactions between genes and environment. But the really exciting news is that the genetic influence, although strong, is not immutable and is readily affected by decisions that you and I make about our parenting.

And I like that.

# 4

# False positives and false negatives

There is much conjecture - in both the scientific literature and the lay press - about the perceived increase in the frequency of the ADHD diagnosis, and the widespread use of stimulant medications. There has in fact been a well-documented surge in prescribing rates of these medications in recent times; for example, it has been estimated that the prevalence of stimulant prescriptions in the US increased fourfold between 1987 and 1996.

High profile figures such as 'Dr Phil' McGraw and Hillary Clinton have added their voices to the growing chorus of concern. If the prevalence of the condition is only supposed to be around six percent, why, in certain schools, does fully half the class take ADHD medication? I have dealt with these schools and their teachers, so I know that it happens.

In the medical and bioethics communities, there is an ongoing vigorous debate about so-called 'cognitive enhancement,' akin to drug use in sport, or cosmetic surgery. Many feel that the stimulants are being inappropriately used for performance enhancement (how else will we get him into an Ivy League university?) rather than properly diagnosed ADHD. Some even argue that there is nothing wrong with using such medications to help with studies if there is no risk involved (a big *if*, I might add). To quote a recently published paper,

> *It is widely recognised that ADHD is over-diagnosed in some affluent communities, where local expectations are such that stimulants are just one more tool to promote performance.*

**But what does the research tell us?**
The Great Smoky Mountain study in the USA provides us with some interesting epidemiological data. In this study, some 1422 children, their parents and their teachers were given structured interviews to ascertain the prevalence of various conditions in the community. The results were quite startling. A mere 57% of the children who had been prescribed stimulant medications actually met criteria for ADHD! Of the entire group who did *not* meet diagnostic criteria for ADHD, as many as 4.5% had received stimulants. In addition, only 72% of those who *did* meet criteria for ADHD were on treatment. We must therefore conclude, if this study is anything to go by, that there is both over-diagnosis (false positives) and under-diagnosis (false negatives) in ADHD.

Let's consider each in turn.

**Conditions which masquerade as ADHD**
The symptoms of ADHD are non-specific; they can occur in a number of other neuropsychiatric conditions. If you experience excessive thirst, pass lots of urine and have wild fluctuations in your blood sugar, it can't be anything other than diabetes (forgive me if you thought of something else; medical school was a long time ago). But if you have poor concentration, you could have, well, just about anything. Indeed, it has been suggested by some that 'ADHD' is nothing other than a final common pathway

for a whole range of insults to the developing brain. Perhaps this is taking it too far, but what it *does* mean, practically, is that we have to think of several possible diagnoses when a child presents with poor concentration.

Take anxiety, for example. It is very common for anxious children to experience poor concentration and restlessness, and to underachieve in the classroom, especially in test situations. It is difficult to focus on the task at hand if you are worrying about something else. You have probably experienced this phenomenon yourself at certain times. Anxiety disorders in childhood are often overlooked in favour of a diagnosis of ADHD.

Similarly, childhood depression is often not recognised as such, partly because it manifests so differently to its adult counterpart. Whilst appetite and sleep disturbances are hallmark features of depression in adults, they often don't feature in childhood depression. But depressed children are often inattentive, unmotivated, easily bored and lethargic, symptoms which are commonly seen in ADHD.

**Childhood bipolar disorder**

There is much controversy about the number of children being diagnosed with Bipolar disorder. This condition shares many symptoms with ADHD, including distractibility, hyperactivity and poor impulse control. Furthermore, ADHD is itself associated with various emotional symptoms, such as low frustration tolerance and irritability, which are commonly seen in Bipolar disorder.

The disagreement is mainly around the diagnostic rules being used for the diagnosis, because again, the accepted adult criteria for Bipolar disorder do not apply to children, at least not to prepubertal children. Generally, the North Americans accept criteria which are broader, resulting in more diagnoses, whereas the British and Europeans favour stricter, tighter rules, resulting in fewer diagnoses.

Psychiatric conditions are sometimes subject to the 'flavour of the month' syndrome. When I was training in child psychiatry, my professor was once moved to issue a temporary ban on the Bipolar diagnosis, in an attempt to help us to see beyond the face-value of presenting symptoms. But whichever side of the transatlantic divide one finds oneself, there is certainly symptom overlap between the two conditions. Furthermore, many children initially thought to have ADHD, later turn out to rather have mood disorders, including (bona fide) Bipolar disorder.

**Learning disorders and executive functions**
A learning disorder is a specific area of weakness in a child's learning profile, out of keeping with his or her overall intellectual ability. This is *not* mental handicap; you can be highly intelligent and yet have a learning disorder. Dyslexia (now called Developmental Reading Disorder) would be an example. Learning disorders and ADHD often mimic each other, largely because they both commonly affect the brain's executive functions, a set of higher order skills which are critical to all of us.

The best analogy I have come across for the executive functions – in Thomas Brown's *Attention Deficit Disorder* – is that of the conductor of an orchestra: the individual players may all be highly skilled, but without an effective conductor, the final product will not be harmonious. Similarly, our executive functions allow us to be productive and effective in the world by harnessing our specific skills, applying each of them in the most efficient manner. A highly intelligent person with poor self-management skills is likely to underachieve. Examples of such skills include planning, prioritising and being able to delay gratification. If you put your hand on your forehead, the brain area on the other side of the bone is the prefrontal cortex (figure 1, chapter 3). Be very thankful for it. This is the part of the brain which helps you to be effective in the world. It is this area which is often faulty in ADHD and in learning disorders. (There are several other conditions which are also associated with poor executive functioning, including Bipolar disorder).

The only way to reliably identify a learning disorder is through an educational assessment, conducted by an appropriately qualified psychologist. Failure to do so can consign a child to unnecessary medications and incorrect school placement, whilst the real issue is ignored. Now, there is no reason why a child can't have both ADHD *and* a learning disorder, and many children do. This brings us to the important topic of comorbidity.

**Comorbidity versus differential diagnosis**
In modern child psychiatry, there is a tendency to diagnose comorbid conditions; that is, several diagnoses co-occurring in the same child. ADHD is often comorbid with a number of other conditions, including those discussed earlier. It is in fact fairly unusual, at least in specialist practice, to see a child with 'pure' ADHD. If we focus only on the ADHD then we run the risk of ignoring important, distressing and impairing symptoms in that child.

The trick is to focus on the most impairing condition first, which may *not* be the ADHD. Then, *if* other symptoms remain and warrant treatment (they may not), we systematically shift our attention to those. This is very important to remember, because otherwise children end up on unnecessary cocktails of medications which may needlessly expose them to nasty side-effects and drug interactions.

But concerns have been raised that our profession is a little too quick to incorporate long lists of comorbid conditions. This was articulated at a recent keynote address I attended by Professor Sir Michael Rutter, arguably the patriarch of child psychiatry. He spoke about the problems inherent in psychiatric classification, and referred to the 'ridiculously high' rate of comorbidity in psychiatry.

Where we have perhaps gone wrong, at least in clinical practice, is that too little attention is now given to the art of *differential diagnosis*, whereby the clinician attempts to ascertain the *single* most likely diagnosis, or at the very least, the most important diagnosis. Without this diagnostic rigour, it is too easy to end up with a long list of conditions in which ADHD invariably features! And worse, it is often treated first when another condition is more of a priority.

**Lessons from the Romanian adoptees**
And now, moving along. We were exploring conditions which masquerade as ADHD. A child's brain is particularly vulnerable to stress. Inattentiveness and overactivity are commonly seen in children who have been subject to emotional and/or physical abuse, and other forms of stress. This would be an example of how the symptoms of ADHD might represent a non-specific 'final common pathway.'

A fascinating and ongoing study is that of the Romanian adoptees, overseen by the same Michael Rutter and his team in England. A group of children from Romanian orphanages were adopted into UK homes after the fall of the Ceaucescu regime in 1989, and have been systematically followed up to date. (This type of study, called a longitudinal study, usually provides more valuable information than a cross-sectional or retrospective study.) These children were exposed to the most abysmal and neglectful early rearing conditions in the first months of their lives. I recently met someone who worked as a volunteer in some of these institutions, and he recalled infants in impossibly cramped conditions, without any stimulation, lying in their own urine and covered in flies.

## A biological programming effect?

Amongst many other problems, this group has an extremely high incidence of overactivity and inattentiveness, much higher than the general population. That may not be too surprising, but a particularly intriguing, perhaps counterintuitive finding, is that the inattentiveness and overactivity in these children did not improve over time, however long they remained in their more nurturing adoptive homes. Closer analysis of the data reveals that the children whose 'dosage' of deprivation prior to adoption was longer than six months, are the ones who are most at risk for a range of negative outcomes, and whose symptoms are static, not showing improvement over time.

This suggests that there seems to be some sort of programming effect on the brain at a critical stage of development, which is very difficult to overcome later on, even in the most nurturing environments. The inference is that the window has shut; the important biological and attachment processes, which we discussed in the previous chapter, occur within a certain time period and then become fixed, or 'hardwired' in. We have already considered insecure attachment as a possible risk factor for ADHD. This study surely adds credence to that hypothesis, although it is difficult to extrapolate from this study – involving children exposed to deprivation of the most severe kind – to the general population.

Many of these adoptees have what is referred to as Reactive Attachment Disorder (RAD), a condition known to result from neglect in infancy, and manifesting with a range of impairments in social functioning. Incidentally, you may be interested to hear that as many as 85% of children with RAD also meet criteria for ADHD, another 'ridiculously high' overlap?

## Adjustment Disorder

And finally on our menu of masqueraders we consider an unfashionable diagnosis. Adjustment Disorder refers to the presence of emotional or behavioural symptoms (including hyperactivity and inattentiveness) occurring within three months of an identifiable stressor in a child's life. We (doctors, teachers and parents) are too quick to overlook this, I fear. Hands up if you've ever heard of it.

If a child's parents have recently separated, and she becomes distractible in class, the correct diagnosis is an Adjustment Disorder, *not* ADHD. Our diagnostic guidelines further stipulate that:

> *once the stressor has terminated, the symptoms do not persist for more than an additional six months.*

If they do persist, then ADHD is on. But what if the stressor *doesn't* terminate, as in the case of an ongoing acrimonious divorce? Do we then retreat behind the safer (and often more acceptable) ADHD label? After all, there is a treatment for it! And a positive response to stimulant medication does not prove the diagnosis of ADHD; it is non-specific. (Indeed, some studies suggest that healthy individuals also derive benefits from stimulant medications). Parents and practitioners alike may pat themselves on the back when the child responds well to such medication, whilst the family issues remain unresolved.

## The folly of medical reductionism

Over-diagnosis can also result from various forms of cognitive bias on the part of doctors and parents alike. As a student, I once failed a clinical exam because of foreclosure. I had prematurely decided what was wrong with the child, and was thus closed to other diagnostic possibilities. This can happen in practice as well. After all, a child is referred by the school, because of academic difficulties, and 'for assessment for ADHD.' There is a risk that the clinician will jump to diagnostic conclusions without considering other causes for the child's concentration difficulties, especially when under time pressure.

A particular error of our age is that of medical reductionism, which refers to the tendency to reduce an inherently complex matter into an overly simplified, one-dimensional 'diagnosis.' Both doctors and parents can fall into this trap, for very different reasons. The doctor, because it is easier and he has a treatment to offer for this diagnosis, and the parents, because they actually prefer a label which lets them off the proverbial hook, rather than implicating their parenting, family lifestyle or worse...

## False negatives

What about the other side of the coin? The

aforementioned Great Smoky Mountain study also highlighted significant *under*-diagnosis, or false negatives: only 72% of those meeting criteria for ADHD actually received treatment. And this was in North America. Elsewhere it is worse. In fact, it has been estimated that world-wide, of all children with mental health needs, as many as 50% don't receive *any* form of treatment.

**Poverty**

When I worked in community clinics in some of the poorest areas of Johannesburg, I was struck by the absence of ADHD referrals. Instead, I was swamped with physical and sexual abuse, foetal alcohol syndrome, the sequelae of HIV/AIDS, abandoned children, and those in need of social grants. My experience is not unique; it seems that the poorer the community, the less likely we are to recognize and treat 'softer' conditions, including ADHD. They are squeezed out by so many more pressing issues; the hierarchy of needs simply hasn't got there yet.

**Gender differences**

In general, girls with ADHD tend to present with less hyperactivity and impulsivity and are less disruptive than their male counterparts. As a consequence, they are far less likely to get up the nose of the teacher, who is, after all, a primary source of referral. Also, girls have a different pattern of comorbidity (you now know what that means). Compared to boys with the condition, they have higher rates of mood and anxiety disorders, which tend to obscure the underlying ADHD. These factors probably explain the well-documented under-identification and under-diagnosis of ADHD in girls.

**Race and ethnicity**
In the United States, it has been documented that Hispanic and African-American children are less frequently diagnosed and treated for ADHD than their white peers. This could be an artifact of affluence and access to healthcare, and this no doubt plays a role, but in at least one study, these differences were independent of socio-economic level. As the authors point out,

> *...important cultural differences exist among persons of diverse ethnic backgrounds with regard to attitudes and beliefs about illness, choice of care, access to care, degree of trust toward authority figures or institutions and tolerances for certain behaviors.*

So as things stand, an African American girl with ADHD from a poor community is unfortunately likely to continue in diagnostic obscurity.

**False positives *and* false negatives**
Is ADHD overdiagnosed? Well, it depends. It depends on your socioeconomic level, your culture, your gender and crucially, your world-view. Inattentiveness in childhood is a non-specific symptom and has to be thoroughly explored in each child. Failure to do so can result in an overly reductionistic assessment which ignores important broader aspects of that child and family, thus neglecting vital areas of intervention. At the same time, ADHD is still widely under-recognised, especially in less affluent areas, where many children are denied potentially life-changing treatment.

# 5

# Prevention is better than cure

ADHD is expensive. Like many chronic conditions, but probably more so than most, it confers a massive burden on society. This burden includes the cost of healthcare, educational underachievement, substance abuse, delinquency and (in adults) loss of work productivity.

Several researchers have attempted to quantify this cost. For example, a study published in 2005 in *Current Medical Research and Opinion,* estimated the healthcare and work loss costs of children and adults with ADHD (treated and untreated) in the United States, by looking at data from a large insurance company. These authors concluded that the total annual *excess* cost (that over and above what would be expected for the general population) was $31.6 billion dollars (roughly equivalent to the GDP of Latvia).

In third world countries (including parts of South Africa), the situation is aggravated by a lack of available resources, including medications and appropriately trained professionals. And if you are lucky enough to have access to treatment, getting it funded by insurers is another uphill battle. If you have a child with ADHD, you have probably experienced this. Furthermore, the currently available treatments, as effective as they can be, have limited impact on longterm outcome; symptoms tend to recur when the intervention is discontinued.

## Can ADHD be prevented?

These factors have prompted the scientific community to turn its attention to the possibility of prevention of ADHD, or at least early intervention, which might alter the course of the condition. Several aspects of the disorder suggest that this might be possible. After all, as we have discovered, it is a developmental condition, which often overlaps with immaturity, and there are a group of children whose symptoms do resolve over time. Also, despite the genetic underpinnings of ADHD, the risk genes are themselves susceptible to environmental influences.

## Primary prevention

The purest type of prevention, known as primary prevention, kicks in before any symptoms are evident and aims to prevent the condition emerging at all, in any form. Education about the dangers of maternal smoking and alcohol in pregnancy, would be one such example. Other preventive strategies have targeted the attachment phase of development.

Through her acclaimed 'Roots of Empathy' programme, educator Mary Gordon has created a strategy which incorporates the important lessons of attachment into the classroom curriculum. In her words,

> *It is to our advantage to have the story of human development taught to all children in school; it fosters universal respect for the fundamental importance of secure first relationships and for the family as the most influential source of all that is truly human.*

Although her focus is not specifically ADHD (or any other condition), the idea – supported by compelling research – is that teaching children about attachment helps to nurture the development of empathy, which will in turn determine how they as adults influence the next generation.

## A window of opportunity

But my vote for the most cost-effective prevention strategy goes to antenatal classes and well-baby clinics. Or at least it would, if they were any good. What better forum to educate new parents (and these days, dads *and* moms attend) about the importance of attachment in the development of their child? I am convinced that if they only knew, we would have far fewer childhood problems generally, and certainly less 'ADHD.' I don't think it is too far-fetched to suggest that society overall would benefit from a more intentional approach to antenatal programmes, possibly even at a public health level. This would also be a very cost-effective intervention.

The developmental psychologist Jay Belsky is one of the more influential researchers in the field of early child development. In 1988 he caused a stir by reporting in *Child Development,* that children exposed to more than 20 hours per week of non-maternal care were more insecurely attached than their peers. This was a very important finding, because insecure attachment, as we have learnt, in turn predicts poorer developmental outcomes. Belsky's study has been dissected and criticised over the years; it seems that several other factors also play a role, including the *quality* of 'non-maternal care.' But the important point is that attachment *matters*, and it all happens in the early months of life.

Whenever I speak to expectant parents on this topic, I

am struck by how receptive they are; and judging by subsequent feedback, this information has influenced their decisions in those critical early months of parenting. They are ready to listen, and they act on the advice they are given. This provides a window of opportunity which we dare not waste. It is far easier to 'set out your stall' the correct way, than to have to rearrange it after the baby arrives, or indeed after the second or third child arrives.

**Turn off the TV**
For 'TV' please read 'electronic screen' (I won't attempt a comprehensive list of all varieties; more will be invented by the time this is published!). In 1999, The American Academy of Paediatrics took the unprecedented step of publicly recommending that children under the age of two should watch no television whatsoever, and thereafter, no more than two hours per day. If the supporting research wasn't quite there at the time, it certainly is now. Whether we consider development generally, or ADHD specifically, there is now good evidence for the damaging effects of TV in the first three years of life.

This shouldn't surprise us. Watching television deprives babies of critical contact time with humans, which will have a direct impact on the quality of their attachment. Also, there is the opportunity cost of missing out on other forms of stimulation, so vital for cognitive development at a time of life when the brain is at its most plastic. One of the hallmark features of ADHD (and arguably modern society) is an inability to wait. Listening to people is usually a waiting situation which requires a degree of patience and self-control. Watching television is exactly the opposite; it is fast, stimulating and immediate.

It would be misleading to suggest that excessive exposure to TV *causes* ADHD, but by now you probably realise that it's naive to speak about any single cause of ADHD. It is a complex, multifaceted condition with many risk factors. Preventive strategies must therefore target these risk factors and so-called 'pathway modifiers,' which alter the trajectory of the condition. TV is one of them.

Some of the other topics which should be covered by any self-respecting antenatal course, would include the following:

- the impact of maternal stress in pregnancy
- the mom-going-back-to-work debate
- the importance of identifying post-natal depression
- engaging with your infant
- the consequences of outsourcing parenting to au-pairs and domestic helpers, especially at this early stage.

As it is, you can learn about the virtues of underwater birth, when to introduce pumpkin, and nappy rashes. I don't mean to sound cynical or anything.

**Targetting genes**
If it were possible, and it isn't (yet), gene therapy would be another example of primary prevention. But that doesn't mean that we have no way of influencing the genome for good. In chapter three the topic of epigenetics was introduced, the phenomenon by which certain genes can be modified by environmental factors, both physical *and* emotional.

There is strong circumstantial evidence implicating epigenetic mechanisms in ADHD. For example, let's consider twins again. If there was a straight line between carrying risk genes and having the condition, we would expect identical twins not to differ with respect to the disorder. But they do, and this variance (we call it *discordance*) cannot be accounted for by environmental factors alone.

As the following data suggests, epigenetic mechanisms are playing a role. In a recent longitudinal study of several twin pairs, it was found that DNA methylation (a major epigenetic mechanism) of several genes, including the 7R variant of the DRD4 gene, differed markedly even in identical twin pairs, from as early as five years old. Furthermore, the methylation pattern was different within individuals, when measured later on at aged ten. These results suggest that the environment plays an important role in the different expression of these genes between individuals and over time.

Much more research is needed, but it is very exciting to think that the choices we make as parents may prevent the emergence of an impairing condition like ADHD.

## What about secondary prevention?

Is it possible to alter the progression or trajectory of the condition *after* symptoms have become evident? The evidence to date suggests that we can. Around ten years ago, the American National Institute of Mental Health (NIMH) funded a large, randomised study, evaluating ADHD treatment in several hundred preschoolers (aged 3 to 6), with severe ADHD. The main aim of the so-called PATS (Preschoolers ADHD Treatment Study) was to research the effects of stimulant medications in this age-group, information which was sorely lacking at the time.

But we are interested in a particular aspect of this study. Prior to entering the medication arm of the trial, all families had to undergo a 10-week parent-training programme, incorporating various behavioural strategies. The children with unsatisfactory improvements in ADHD symptom severity following parent-training, proceeded to drug treatment.

As it turned out, the parenting strategies were so effective that as many as 30% of these children no longer warranted medication at all, or their parents were satisfied enough with their progress to withdraw them from the next phase. This is a very important (and often overlooked) finding, providing evidence that early intervention can improve matters significantly. But can it have a more lasting effect on the trajectory of the condition? We probably don't have the answers yet, but we are starting to see some interesting work, like that of Jeff Halperin and his team, to which we now turn our attention.

**The benefits of Hopscotch**
A psychiatrist based in New York, Halperin has a particular interest in early intervention in ADHD. At a recent conference in Barcelona, he presented the results of an experiment in which four and five year old children with ADHD were enrolled in a programme of environmental stimulation.

The theory goes like this. We know that ADHD is a developmental condition, and that it resolves in several children. If we can harness the brain mechanism(s) by which it resolves, and intentionally incorporate these into our interventions, then we should be able to facilitate symptom resolution. This team turned its attention to the proven benefits to the developing brain of exercise and cognitive stimulation. Furthermore, the best way to deliver this stimulation is in a social context, rather than behind a computer screen. Several decades ago, the term 'scaffolding' was coined, to describe the process by which more knowledgeable people try to help less knowledgeable ones, to enable them to learn new concepts or skills. It comprises several key components, not the least of which is the emotional connection between the teacher and learner. As a parent, you are that 'more knowledgeable person.'

So with that theoretical background, Halperin's team set up a programme including games such as 'Simon Says,' The Memory Game and Hopscotch, each one carefully chosen for its developmental value. Parents were to perform a set of such tasks with their children for 30-45 minutes daily, for at least five days per week, over the duration of the study. Notably, it didn't have to be with the child alone, but could be done as a family-based activity. Compliance (or *adherence,* as we say these days) was good; there was no problem getting families to do this, as there often is with medication, or even other behavioural interventions.

And the results were highly encouraging. A significant improvement in ADHD symptoms was evident, even based on teacher feedback (remember it was the parents giving the intervention). The beauty of this approach is that it uses everyday life and is easily implemented, without much cost or training. We all do these things anyway with our kids, or at least we *should.* But the really exciting part of this study is that the benefits were sustained long after the study was discontinued, as long as twelve months, according to the paper. I can only imagine that many families continued with the programme, having been pointed in the right direction. It beats watching TV.

What this study can't tell us, however, is *why* these children improved. The likely possibilities include enhanced neural development as hypothesized earlier, or perhaps the benefits were mediated by an improvement in the parent-child relationship. It could even be both. Now, as Halperin himself admitted, this was not a randomised trial; in other words, there was no control group receiving another form of intervention against which the effects could be compared, to give the research more statistical clout. So the next step is to do exactly that.

And I, for one, await those results with eager anticipation.

# 6

# Dietary strategies for ADHD

## (and other ineffective treatments)

Not too long ago, the South African government famously advocated a diet of beetroot and sweet potatoes as a treatment for HIV/AIDS. It really did. To our acute national embarrassment, the South African stand at the World HIV Conference in Toronto in 2006 consisted of an assortment of vegetables; an antiretroviral drug was not to be seen (until later, as an afterthought).

This is perhaps an extreme example, but illustrative nonetheless. When influential people (and governments) mislead us, people suffer unnecessarily. It costs lives. In the field of ADHD the stakes are perhaps not as high, but society still pays a price for misinformation. Unnecessary suffering, delays in treatment and expense all result from misguided policies.

Trawling our way through all the quackery also has the unfortunate effect of distracting us from more productive endeavours. You should minimise junk food, fizzy drinks and sweets, for several reasons. But you didn't need me to tell you that. A balanced diet is necessary and good, and we need to pay attention to it, especially since there is now a well-documented association between ADHD and childhood obesity (itself an international health emergency). But instead, we end up spending our energies fending off the spurious claims of self-professed nutritional experts. This is the opportunity cost of all the hype around ADHD. We are in danger of neglecting common sense amidst all the pseudoscientific wonder cures.

But if your child has ADHD, you will unfortunately need to do some trawling. Relevant scientific findings in any field, especially in health, should not be the sole preserve of eccentric university professors, shrouded in mystery and beyond the reach of the average layperson. You, the concerned parent, have both a right and an obligation to know the facts. You will not find them in the newspaper or on TV. Nor, sadly, will you find them in the average doctor's consultation. But they are knowable.

Let's begin.

**'Vitamins are more natural than Ritalin; they must therefore be a better treatment for ADHD.'**

How do we know that a treatment works? As correct as a remedy might *seem*, the only way to know if it works is to properly test it. Anecdotal report cannot be trusted, and nor can intuition. Have a look at figure 3:

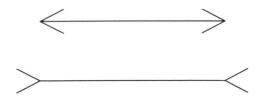

**Figure 3**

Which line is longer? They are in fact the same length, but if you trusted your intuition, you would be wrong. This is an example of a visual illusion, but we are also susceptible to many cognitive illusions, as shown by the likes of Nobel prizewinning researcher and writer Daniel Kahnemann. This is why we measure things, which is what the scientific method is all about.

**A fair test**

Let's say I wanted to prove that high dose Vitamin C is an effective treatment for ADHD. The first step is to collect a group of kids reliably diagnosed with the condition. The group must be large enough to provide meaningful results. I then randomly split them into two groups, one which receives the tested treatment, and another (the control group) which takes fake Vitamin C pills. The fake pills are the placebo, a 'treatment' which doesn't contain the active ingredient – in this example, ascorbic acid – but is in other respects indistinguishable; it looks, tastes and feels the same, and is administered in the same way.

After a reasonable time period, say four weeks, I measure how each group has done (using an accepted rating scale) and compare their progress. This forms the basis of the randomised placebo-controlled trial, which is the gold-standard in testing proposed treatments for any medical condition.

It's not rocket science, it's just science.

**Publication bias**

Having completed my experiment, it is very important that I publish my findings, *whether positive or negative*. A negative study is not a bad study but one in which the tested treatment failed to beat placebo. As such, it provides useful information (much more than a bad positive study), but unfortunately many negative studies are never published. This is called *publication bias*, and there are several reasons for it. It is human nature, after all, to prefer positive to negative findings; they are more exciting. It is also disquieting that big pharmaceutical companies are sometimes guilty of publication bias; their agenda is to register their product, and negative studies just won't do.

Doctors make decisions involving the lives of their patients based on this published literature. If I only publish the one positive trial, and quietly bin the ones which failed to show benefits, I am misleading the public and my colleagues, sometimes scandalously so.

## Replicating results

And if my study was positive, and I go around claiming that high dose Vitamin C treats ADHD, my colleagues and the public need access to the methodology I used, and how I came to my conclusions. Otherwise my claims will rightly be treated with suspicion. If this is really going to be a breakthrough treatment, my findings will need to be replicated by others; this is impossible if I don't publish them for all to see.

## Meta-analysis

Publication also allows other authors to re-examine my data at a later date, using other statistical methods. If we have ten small trials all independently conducted, it is often possible to lump them all together to make one big trial, thus improving the value of the data. This is called a meta-analysis, and is a very important methodological tool. Trials are often expensive to conduct, and thus often include smaller patient numbers than would be ideal. Meta-analysis can overcome this. But a word of caution is in order here. It is possible to 'doctor' a meta-analysis, by only including the trials which suit your purpose. This is referred to as *cherrypicking,* and it is unfortunately a common occurrence in the field.

Now, most purported remedies for ADHD have not even been subjected to proper testing (despite what their proponents might claim); for these, all that can be concluded is that they *may* work, but we just don't know yet. So the next time you are told by a nutritionist or homeopath that their remedy has been tested, you have some clarifying questions of your own to ask:

### How many patients were tested?
If the numbers are too low, then it is unlikely for a putative treatment to pass the statistical test of efficacy. If five patients out of seven get better, that doesn't tell me much, but 500 out of 700 should make me sit up and take notice. A small trial might still be included in a meta-analysis, but then again we need to be vigilant to the possibility of cherrypicking.

### Was a proper placebo arm used?
This is very important, because placebo has been found to work quite well, especially in children. Our attitudes to treatment, it seems, have a very powerful effect. The *Hawthorne* effect is a related and well-known research phenomenon, whereby symptoms improve simply because they are being scrutinised. If I focus on your impulse control for four weeks, it is likely to improve, whatever treatment I give you. So if I want to prove that my treatment works, I need to show that it beats placebo.

### How were the patients chosen?
For a test to be fair, those who receive the treatment and

those who get placebo need to be randomly chosen. Otherwise, as ethical as the researcher might consider himself, he is open to bias as to who gets included where. For example, knowing that Mr Jones is a patient who is never satisfied no matter what I do, I might slip him into the placebo group, lest he spoil my results!

### *Who did the measuring?*

Another pitfall in many trials is the lack of proper blinding when results are measured. After four weeks of treatment, those who do the measuring should be unaware of who is taking the actual Vitamin C and who is taking the placebo. Otherwise, the prejudices of those conducting the trial (we are all subject to them) may influence their recording of the results. This has been well documented; without proper blinding, there is an increased likelihood of a trial yielding a falsely positive result.

### *What was the duration of the trial?*

The shorter the duration (say only a week of high dose Vitamin C), the less reliable my findings. One of the reasons for this, is what we call *regression to the mean*. When your flu is at its worst, you go to the doctor, who prescribes an antibiotic and you start to improve. You erroneously conclude that the pills made you better, when all that really happened, is that your flu started to improve anyway. There is a natural ebb and flow of symptoms in most illnesses, including chronic conditions. To overcome this (and for other reasons), we need to test treatments for long enough.

### Diet and ADHD

Thus armed, let's examine the evidence for some commonly advocated ADHD remedies, starting with diet.

We begin with the restricted, or elimination diet. The theory behind this approach is that some children have food intolerances or allergies, which aggravate their symptoms. If these foodstuffs can be identified and eliminated, inattentiveness and hyperactivity should improve.

Two large studies of elimination diets did show improvements in ADHD symptoms, but they were not blinded, and so (as you now know) have to be taken with a pinch of salt. Of those which were blinded, the majority did not show significant benefits, except when children were carefully selected for food intolerances.

Perhaps worthy of special mention is a randomised, placebo-controlled trial of 100 ADHD kids in the Netherlands (did you nod approvingly three times?), published in 2011 in the *Lancet*. These researchers began by eliminating everything but rice, meat, vegetables, pears and water, and saw who improved. Those who did were then systematically challenged to identify which foods aggravated their symptoms, and their diets were tailored accordingly. Of this subgroup, several children experienced significant symptomatic improvement.

In other words, the restricted diet approach does work for some children. But the catch is that you have to properly identify who those children are (a minority of ADHD kids), a time-consuming and expensive process requiring expert supervision. Overall, the improvements are small, far smaller than the effects we get with medication. But, of course, this is a safe treatment, and free of the side-effects associated with prescription drugs.

So restriction diets cannot, at this stage, be advocated wholesale, but in certain children they probably play a role.

**Artificial food colourants**

The widespread use of artificial food colourants in modern diets has been blamed by some for the explosion of ADHD diagnoses, and the increase in stimulant prescriptions. The azo-dyes in particular (such as tartrazine), have been the subject of investigation for the past 40 years. But the studies examining the benefits of excluding these compounds have also been blighted by poor methodology, such as parental reports rather than blinded measurements. Overall, the evidence is less than convincing.

**The fish oils**

There is some theoretical rationale for using the omega-3 fatty acids (in products such as Eye-q and Equazen) in ADHD. These 'essential fatty acids' (essential because they aren't produced by the body, they have to be ingested) are important structural components of cell membranes, especially in the brain. Several studies have demonstrated differences in omega-3 fatty acid composition in patients with ADHD compared with unaffected controls. Also, these compounds can indirectly affect dopamine activity, a neurotransmitter which is known to be involved in the symptoms of ADHD.

Wading through the published studies on the topic (I didn't but I'm very thankful that someone did), we find ten which pass methodological muster, involving a total of 699 patients. A recently published meta-analysis (pooling together) of these studies, revealed a small but significant improvement in ADHD symptoms. The caveat here is that the dosage has to be high enough, otherwise don't bother. Again, the effect is small compared to established medications, but given their benign side-effect profile, the authors conclude (and I agree with them) that they could be used to augment traditional drug treatment, or in families who refuse prescribed medications.

## All the other stuff

From there, it just gets worse. When flawed trials are excluded, neurofeedback, homeopathy, various forms of cognitive training and even several behavioural treatments all flop. If you really insist, I can go on to mention brain gym, Bach flower remedies, heavy metal chelation, reiki, reflexology, energy rebalancing, colonic irrigation and the like. But I think you've got the point.

Now, can we please move on?

# 7

# What's the fuss about medication?

It has been said that we live in a chemically complacent society. Neuroscience has taken giant forward strides in recent decades, and it is this very medical progress, coupled with modern society's constant demand for the 'quick fix,' which have brought us face to face with the thorny issue of medicating psychological symptoms in children. I have met parents on both sides of the ideological divide. I have been frustrated by parental unwillingness to consent to medication, when their children are clearly suffering as a result of treatable conditions, which could well have a significant impact on their development. I have also found myself in the perhaps more uncomfortable position of feeling coerced into prescribing medication, when I have not been convinced that it was in the best interests of the child.

It seems to me that in the field of medicine, there are few more emotive issues than this one. This is important to acknowledge, because emotions can distort our thinking. No parent takes kindly to negative feedback of any sort about their child. We are naturally defensive about our offspring. When a teacher declares that a child 'should go onto Ritalin,' as often happens, one can understand how this suggestion will be met with parental resistance.

Also, we must not forget that we are dealing with minors, who are inherently vulnerable. It thus behoves us, as adults, to be extremely cautious about using medication which interacts with their still-developing brains, however well-researched the medication might be. Would you not agree that there is something basically counterintuitive about using pills to treat psychological and behavioural problems? It somehow *feels* wrong. Whether or not it is rational to feel this way, I don't know. Perhaps our collective conscience is telling us something. But whatever the reasons, controversy abounds.

**The meaning of a symptom**
A headache might be telling us a number of things: dehydration, too much time behind the computer, psychological stress, meningitis, to name but a few. The solution is not necessarily a pill - although it might provide symptomatic relief - but to investigate the underlying reason and then treat that. Indeed, such symptomatic relief may even be dangerous, masking the condition and delaying the identification and proper treatment of the true diagnosis.

Similarly, in the field of psychiatry, we have to consider the underlying meaning of a psychological symptom. A child might experience debilitating anxiety for several reasons. If her mother is an alcoholic, then the priority must be to address the parent's condition, which will almost certainly alleviate the child's symptoms (although it may take a little longer). Prescribing medication for this child, whilst neglecting the pathology in the family, could do more harm than good, at least in the medium to long term. And it is this potential trap that I believe to be the greatest danger in prescribing psychoactive medication for children.

There are several contemporary influences contributing to our 'quick-fix' culture. We have already considered medical reductionism, the tendency to oversimplify complex clinical problems. A child with severe tantrums might be diagnosed as Oppositional Defiant Disorder: a neat, clear-cut diagnosis. The true state of affairs may be far more complicated, involving, for example, principles of discipline or the father's own temper. I have interviewed many children who are aware (at least at some level) that they are being made the presenting symptom of a dysfunctional family system, and are justifiably angry at the hypocrisy it represents.

Make no mistake, it is not only doctors who fall prey to this trap; it is a societal phenomenon, pervading our thinking, and touching many other disciplines besides medicine. Many parents and indeed teachers tend to seek out a diagnostic label rather than facing up to their own role in the child's symptoms, or the management thereof. Even the system of medical aid reimbursement encourages this oversimplification of inherently complex issues. Unless I attach a label, my patient will not get reimbursed: 'complex family issues and alcoholic father' won't fly.

**The role of the media**
In *Bad Science*, Ben Goldacre laments the current state of medical journalism, arguing that the quality of such reporting has deteriorated markedly, due to the declining number of dedicated medical journalists. This results in a misinterpretation of scientific findings, and a misinformed public. There are some notable examples of how unbalanced media reporting has caused considerable harm to public health, not the least of which is the MMR hoax. Some dubious research, carried on the wings of emotive reporting, erroneously linked the Measles/Mumps/Rubella

vaccine to the development of autism, leading to a surge in these quite debilitating yet preventable infections.

The media tends to sensationalise rather than provide a balanced (more boring?) account of an issue. There is a silent majority of children and families for whom ADHD medication is life-changing, but these stories don't seem to be heard; perhaps they are less newsworthy? After all, the business of the media is selling news. And of course, anyone can post anything on the internet. In countries like the United States, where the pharmaceutical industry can market directly to the public, the media can of course contribute to a *pro*-medication bias, so it runs both ways. What this all means is that you, the consumer, need to be correctly appraised of the facts.

So here we go.

**Medications for ADHD and how they work**

Broadly speaking, there are two groups of ADHD medications available to us: the stimulants and the non-stimulants. Stimulants include Ritalin and Concerta - the active ingredient of both being methylphenidate - and the amphetamines, such as Adderall and Dexedrine. The sole representative from the non-stimulant class is Strattera, whose active ingredient is atomoxetine.

Now you will need to cast your mind back to the neuroscience tutorial in chapter three. These drugs all work in areas of the brain known to be affected in ADHD, including the prefrontal cortex and the cerebellum, and pathways emanating from them (figure 1). The stimulants work by blocking the dopamine transporter protein (figure 2), thus increasing the availability of the dopamine neurotransmitter in the synapse. This has the effect of increasing the message transmission from neuron A to neuron B, and hence facilitating the firing of brain circuits. Thus the medication 'kickstarts' certain key pathways which are dysfunctional in the condition. As a result of these chemical events, symptoms resolve.

And they really *do* resolve. Numerous well-designed, randomised, placebo-controlled studies attest to this. But the catch is that symptoms only resolve whilst the medication is active; when it wears off, they recur. Ritalin often needs to be given several times a day, as it only lasts about four hours per dose. There are longer acting stimulants, which alleviate this problem. Ritalin LA (long-acting) lasts 6-8 hours per dose, and Concerta around 10 hours. But none of the stimulants lasts a full 24 hour cycle.

Strattera works in a similar way, but it preferentially increases noradrenaline availability in the synaptic space. The advantage of Strattera is that it has a 24 hour duration of action. This eliminates the need for top-up dosages, and provides an effect at certain key times of the day, such as the early morning getting-ready-for-school routine, when the symptoms of ADHD can be particularly problematic (you can probably think of other adjectives!). Other advantages of Strattera include its benefits in anxiety, and its safety in children with tic disorders (involuntary muscle twitches), such as Tourette's Disorder.

But generally the first choice medication for ADHD would be one of the stimulants, because they are more likely to work. In psychiatry we make a big deal about something called the 'effect size' of a medication. The higher the effect size, the greater the likelihood of it being effective for a given diagnosis. An effect size of 1 would mean perfection, that the medication works in 100% of individuals with that condition. The stimulants have impressively high effect sizes, around 0.8, which is about as good as you can get in psychiatry, and probably in medicine generally. Strattera's is a little lower (although this has been challenged by some).

Other medications having reasonable levels of evidence in ADHD include extended release clonidine and extended release guanfacine; neither of these are currently registered in South Africa (although the short-acting version of clonidine is available). Your child may have been prescribed yet other medications, but they are almost always used to treat comorbid (co-existing) conditions.

## The safety profile of ADHD medications

Understandably, the greatest concern of parents is around the physical safety of prescribed medications. There are certainly a number of possible side-effects, and careful monitoring is required in all cases. If you read the package insert (and by all means do), you will encounter a bewildering array of possible problems with the drug. But remember that the same is true for paracetamol, and it is a legal requirement for the manufacturer to declare everything that has ever happened to anyone, anywhere, on this medication. It's like the small print in an insurance contract: it has to be there, but if you become too obsessed with it, you will remain uninsured.

In practice, I usually only warn parents about five or six side-effects, but I will use my discretion. For example, if there is a family history of tics, then I will tell parents that this is a potential side-effect with the stimulants. Otherwise I probably won't mention it. Many side-effects are transient, including stomach aches and headaches, which are usually alleviated by the child having a good breakfast with the medication, and remaining well hydrated.

## Growth concerns

Loss of appetite can be more troublesome. Some children lose weight on these medications, or fail to gain weight as they should. This tends to be more of an issue with the longer acting drugs which affect the appetite for more of the day. A healthy breakfast is particularly important for children taking these agents, as it is the one meal of the day which can't be affected by appetite suppression (provided, of course, the drug is taken *after* breakfast, which it should be). Thus a very important aspect of monitoring is to regularly check the weight and height of the child. Of course, for some children, a little weight loss may be quite welcome.

Over time, the rate of growth of a child can also be affected. This is highly individual, but overall, the average reduction in height gain is around one centimetre per year, over the first three years of treatment. In certain children, who experience a marked slowdown in growth, we have to come up with another plan, or sometimes even discontinue the treatment.

But I'm sure you will agree that a more critical issue is whether or not there is any impact on *final* adult height. The available evidence suggests that this is not the case and that there is later catch-up growth, although longer duration and better quality studies are needed. In any event, faced with the alternative of academic underachievement, social isolation and a chronically low self-esteem, I may be prepared to sacrifice a centimetre or so. How about you?

## Effects on the heart

During the period January 1992 to February 2005, twenty-eight childhood cases of sudden death during treatment with stimulants were reported. This caused (and continues to cause) a storm of controversy. What we must remember, though, is that twelve of these children had pre-existing structural heart conditions. Furthermore, the estimated rates of sudden death based on these reports is actually *below* background rates of sudden death in the general population. Nonetheless, since both the stimulants and non-stimulants can increase blood pressure and pulse rate, it is important to monitor these parameters both at baseline and during treatment. In addition, we need to be extremely cautious of using these agents in children with pre-existing heart defects, a history of chest pain at rest, heart palpitations or fainting spells, or for whom there is a family history of sudden unexplained death.

## 'Kiddie Cocaine: Behavior Drug Ritalin Abused by Children'

Headlines such as this one (CBS news, February 11th 2009) have justifiably shocked parents worldwide. Let's examine this claim and its implications. What is it actually trying to say?

Could it mean, Ritalin is addictive like cocaine? It isn't. This is because methylphenidate, unlike cocaine, has very little effect on the *nucleus accumbens*, the area of the brain which mediates euphoria and substance dependence. The *rate* of uptake into the brain is critical here. Taken orally, Ritalin gets there too slowly to affect this part of the brain. If you take the time and trouble to crush methylphenidate tablets, and then snort or inject the powder, you can certainly induce euphoria, but prescribed in therapeutic doses and taken correctly, you don't get high on Ritalin.

Could it mean, Ritalin will increase the risk of later drug abuse? It won't. The overwhelming message from the scientific literature is that neither ADHD nor its treatment has much bearing at all on the likelihood of eventual substance abuse. The most important factor influencing the risk for later drug abuse is the presence of conduct disorder. If anything, stimulant treatment into adolescence is actually *protective* against this outcome, probably because of reduced impulsiveness, better social functioning and improvements in self-esteem, which have all been independently shown to minimise the risk of drug abuse.

Could it mean, Ritalin wrecks lives like cocaine? It doesn't. There is a wealth of research which attests to the positive outcomes of those appropriately treated with ADHD medication. In whichever domain you care to mention, be it academic, social, emotional or interpersonal, this treatment enhances the quality of life of those who need it.

So what *does* it mean? Is there a grain of truth in this analogy? On a neurochemical level, both substances affect the dopamine transporter, which controls the amount of dopamine available in the synapse between cells. They both block it, resulting in an increase in the available dopamine (albeit in different parts of the brain). But this is about the extent of the similarity.

Like me, you may have experienced the sense of wellbeing derived from cardiovascular exercise. It is well documented that a good workout results in the release of naturally-occurring *endorphins*, which interact with specific receptors in the brain, causing a mild euphoria. This explains why some long-distance runners get 'addicted' to their exercise. As it turns out, opioid drugs such as morphine and heroin act on the very same brain receptors. Surely you will not use this coincidence of chemistry to condemn my exercise habits?

## Diversion

That said, we do now wade into murkier waters. There certainly is justifiable concern over the phenomenon of diversion, whereby stimulant medications are sought by high school and university students for the wrong purposes. Research conducted in the United States suggests that among college students who are treated with prescription stimulants for ADHD, a majority are approached to sell, trade, or give away their medication each year. I have had patients give me similar feedback about this trend on South African campuses. These medications are sought for their alerting properties, to be used as a study aid, and also sometimes to attain euphoria.

I have also learnt to be cautious of stimulant abuse by parents of my patients; mothers in particular may abuse these drugs to lose weight. The take-home message is that tight control over prescribing is particularly important with this class of medication (as you have no doubt discovered if your child happens to be taking one of these agents). This potential for abuse, although small and limited to certain age-groups, is where Strattera may offer an advantage over the stimulant medications.

## Psychological dependence

Another potential risk is the *psychological* dependence that might follow from a laissez-faire approach to medications. As much as I love my children, there are times in the evenings when I am quite desperate for them to sleep. Simply having an uninterrupted conversation with my wife is a near impossibility until this part of the evening routine is successfully negotiated. My eldest is a night-owl and battles to wake up in the mornings; her natural sleep-wake cycle is just set up that way. These days, we say she has 'Delayed Sleep Phase Disorder.'

There is even a treatment for this condition, in the form of melatonin. And it gets even better, as no script is required (at least in South Africa), and I don't even need to feel parental guilt, since it is a natural hormone, secreted by the brain's pineal gland. So why then have I not resorted to melatonin? What's there to lose?

If it were not for the experience of private practice, I may well have resorted to it. But over the years I have seen several children who, having been successfully started on melatonin, after a time don't believe they can sleep without it. This becomes a self-fulfilling prophesy, and we end up with a child who is psychologically dependent on pills. It is not a tendency I wish to foster in the developing personality of a child, mine or anyone else's. There has to be sufficient impairment due to the condition in question, to warrant a trial of medication, *even* an over-the-counter medication. In my daughter there isn't.

**Emotional effects of ADHD medications**
I routinely warn parents about the potential emotional side-effects of ADHD medications. This may take the form of a subduing effect, and when people talk about their child being a 'zombi' on such medication, this is probably what they mean. Vulnerable children may even become morbid and depressed, some voicing suicidal thoughts. Typically, this tends to occur in children who have a genetic vulnerability to depression (a family member has had it). As you will recall from chapter four, undetected depression can sometimes masquerade as ADHD, and an emotional reaction to an ADHD medication often serves as the unmasking event.

**Suicidal thinking**

In 2005, the US Food and Drug Administration (FDA) issued a 'black box warning' to the product labelling of Strattera, due to the emergence of a small but significant increased incidence of 'suicide related events' in children taking this drug, compared to those on placebo.

I have seen this side-effect in my practice with both atomoxetine and the stimulants, but I do think we are in danger of over-reacting to this warning. In research parlance, 'suicide-related events' include not only suicide attempts, but also suicidal thoughts and even transient beliefs in the pointlessness of life (which would probably include me, on Mondays). More importantly, in the big studies of both atomoxetine and the stimulants, no completed suicides were reported, and the vast majority of 'events' were of mild and transient symptoms that did not require hospitalisation.

Furthermore, ADHD is *itself* associated with an increased risk of suicidality - often due to comorbid conditions such as depression - so it should not be automatically assumed that suicidal thinking in a child with ADHD is necessarily due to his or her treatment. And finally, we must remember that deliberate self-harm (suicidal behaviour) is actually quite common in the general population. Indeed, population-based studies reveal an overall incidence no less than that associated with ADHD medications.


**Rebound effects**

Another emotional side-effect, commoner with short-acting Ritalin, is so-called *rebound* emotionality. This occurs when the medication is wearing off at the end of a dose, and is often aggravated by the lack of food intake in the preceding hours. We try to overcome this by ensuring adequate eating at school break-times, but this is usually easier said than done. It is also often helpful to provide a snack in the car on the way home from school, to deal with the aggravating effect of the sugar low.

## Emotional benefits

Finally, I should also mention that many children on treatment experience emotional *improvements*. They experience more positive feedback from parents and teachers alike, and hence self-esteem improves. They are less anxious about school and enjoy it more. Extramural activities are more rewarding because they can concentrate on what the coach is saying. Overall, these children are usually happier on their medication than off it.

## The medication trial

There is no way of knowing in advance whether a particular medication will be effective for a given child, even with the most accurate diagnosis. Hence we refer to a 'trial' of medication. Parents are often disappointed and frustrated when the first medication is unsuccessful, because of ineffectiveness or side-effects, or both, and give up on the process prematurely. There is usually an effective, well-tolerated alternative. If a child's symptoms continue to cause significant impairment, it is worth continuing systematically until the correct medication is found, even if this requires a second opinion. Unfortunately, whilst we await more sophisticated biological markers of brain function, there remains a trial-and-error aspect to the prescribing process.

In my experience, very few parents of children with concentration difficulties have not heard of at least one 'horror story' involving medications used for ADHD.

In our consumer-driven society, there must always be someone or something to blame. And medication provides a very convenient scapegoat for almost anything which can go wrong with a child. In many instances, far too much is attributed to adverse drug effects than is actually the case. There are certainly occasions of horrible, distressing side-effects, and I have no wish to trivialise these. But it is incorrect to extrapolate from one child's experience to another, and the only way to know how *your* child will respond is to commence a trial, with appropriate monitoring.

The duration of the medication trial is typically four weeks. In that time, the task of the doctor is to ascertain, firstly, whether or not the treatment has been effective in alleviating the target symptoms, and secondly, if the child has tolerated it. If both boxes are ticked, then the treatment should continue, albeit with monitoring and fine-tuning of the dosage over time.

Even if your child does experience side-effects, it must be stressed that these are reversible; they will disappear once the medication is discontinued. Of course, you might decide, in collaboration with the specialist, that the potential risks outweigh the potential benefits of such a trial, and that is also fine, provided you have been given all the information.

**The risk-benefit ratio**

And here we arrive at another important concept. What the *risk-benefit ratio* means, is that at any point in the prescribing process, the benefits of the medication must outweigh the side-effects and risks. If not, it must be stopped. For example, if a child is only slightly impaired by his absentmindedness, and experiences severe emotional side-effects on medication, then, I'm sure you will agree, the benefits of continuing that drug do not outweigh the risks. This is a dynamic assessment and can change over time, as he gets older, as his circumstances change, or for a host of other reasons.

## What do I tell my child about the medication?

Parents are often at a loss as to how to communicate this news to their child. They are concerned about the effects on her already bruised self-esteem of yet another negative message. In my experience, feedback about the diagnosis and treatment is often met by the child with relief and excitement; she more than anyone, wants to overcome her symptoms. But the language of this communication will depend on the developmental stage of the child. In early childhood, it is best to avoid technical terms, which she will not properly grasp, but also because we should be cautious of labelling a child whose condition might resolve with maturity. Nor, in your explanation, do you need to highlight your child's deficiencies; it is quite adequate to stress the potential *benefits* of the proposed treatment, in terms she will understand.

As adolescence approaches, it is appropriate to engage with your child around the diagnosis and treatment and what these entail. At this age, she should participate in her treatment decisions. But this is usually a *process* rather than a discrete event, and most parents successfully use their intuition as a guide; you know your child. Probably the worst approach is to cast a veil of secrecy over the condition and the treatment, as unfortunately happens in many families. This is at best unhelpful for your child, and in many cases aggravates the sense of shame she already feels. Don't make it worse for her.

## What about weekends and holidays?

And now we consider a special kind of holiday, called a *drug holiday*. No, it's not what you're thinking; a drug holiday is simply a medication-free period, usually over weekends or school holidays. Strattera has to be given daily, otherwise it won't work properly at all. As far as the stimulants are concerned, the perceived wisdom in the past was to omit them on non-school days. Most modern guidelines, however, recommend continuous use, apart from exceptional circumstances. This is due to increasing awareness of the impairing effects of ADHD in *all* settings, including the home, as well as the social dysfunction associated with the condition.

But it is an individualised decision, and in my practice, many children do have drug holidays. Others might take a lower dosage on weekends and holidays, in order to minimise side-effects but still maintain some continuity of treatment. If there is significant appetite suppression, accompanied by weight loss or concerns about growth, as contemplated earlier, then medication-free days allow for food intake to catch up. Also, if a child's ADHD symptoms are mainly evident at school, as happens in some children, then it may not be necessary to medicate on weekends.

But before we leave this topic, let's have a look at an educational study quoted by Malcolm Gladwell in *Outliers*. The aim of this research, conducted by the sociologist Karl Alexander, was to better understand the so-called 'achievement gap,' whereby children from wealthier homes tend to outperform their less fortunate peers in the classroom. Standardised measures of reading and mathematics were repeatedly performed on 650 American children over a five year period, from first through fifth grade. The researchers assessed the children at two key points annually, in June before the summer vacation, and in September at the beginning of the new school year. They then analysed the results for high, middle and low income groups.

At the outset, in grade one, there were no significant scholastic differences between the socio-economic groups. But over time, as predicted, the more affluent children pulled away, opening up a significant gap by age ten or eleven. The really interesting finding, however, was the comparison between the scores at different points in the year.

In the September through June period – nine months of mostly term time – there was very little difference in relative progress between the groups. All the action, it turns out, was happening between June and September. The children from wealthier homes actually *improved* in their reading and maths over the summer holidays, whereas the poorer kids stagnated. This difference in progress over the *vacation* fully accounted for the cumulative achievement gap between the socioeconomic groups, over several years. The authors (and Gladwell himself) present several possible reasons for this finding, notably the different parental approach to learning seen in wealthier versus poorer homes.

Now, before we get carried away, this was not specifically a study of ADHD children, but what it does tell us, amongst other things, is that *what happens in the holidays is important*. Children don't stop learning when they are not at school.

### For how long will he need to take the treatment?

This is a question I am often asked: 'Will he ever be able to come off it?' In twelve years of clinical practice, I have

78

never had a child become physiologically dependent on an ADHD medication (although, as mentioned, a few mothers have). There is almost no euphoric effect at standard dosages, and no craving for it. But please do not confuse dependence with the ongoing need to take medication for a chronic condition. A diabetic may take insulin for life, as this is a chronic condition; likewise, a child with ADHD may also require medication for many years, but this is not because of physiological dependence. We now know that ADHD is not restricted to childhood. Several good studies show that it persists into adulthood in at least 60% of cases, and so it should not surprise us that many continue to take their medication through college and beyond.

However, the analogy between ADHD and other chronic medical conditions is not a perfect one. ADHD is a developmental condition, it often overlaps with immaturity, and the child's environment influences his symptoms. Due to these factors, many children *do* successfully come off their medication. Usually we would wait at least a year or two before attempting discontinuation, as it takes time for improvements to become entrenched. But if the child is doing well, the accepted approach is to cautiously reduce medication and observe how he does. This again involves trial and error; there is no more scientific way of knowing when the time is right for any given child.

**A double-edged sword**
We must carefully consider the question in every case: would the use of this medication, at this time, enhance the healthy development and improve the overall functioning of this child and his or her family? If medication is used to alleviate inconvenient symptoms, whilst important

parenting principles or lifestyle factors are ignored, then I do a disservice by prescribing. If, on the other hand, medication is an adjunct to a comprehensive, holistic treatment plan, then I feel more comfortable with it, knowing that the correct medication can even facilitate other therapeutic interventions.

Like many scientific advances, the advent of effective psychoactive medications represents a double-edged sword: used indiscriminately, without proper monitoring, it can do more harm than good; used responsibly, for the right child, it can be a Godsend.

# 8

# Parenting a child with ADHD

*There is no fear in love. But perfect love drives out fear, because fear has to do with punishment.*

St John's first letter,
chapter 4, verse 18

Parenting is a great leveller. In practice, parents often ask me if I have my own children, and 'if he were *your* child, would you put him on medication?' I can see why. Head knowledge is helpful, but on the common ground of parenthood, we all understand and speak the same language. Here we are equal. In fact, I'm quite sure that being a father has helped my practice more than my degree has helped my parenting.

To my knowledge, none of my four children has ADHD, so when I speak or write about this topic it is only partially from experience. My contention, though, is that parenting a child with ADHD is not fundamentally different to parenting *any* child. After all, we are dealing with a developmental condition, whose symptoms are seen in the general population and overlap with immaturity. It shouldn't surprise us. The principles are the same, it's just that the stakes are higher; it matters more.

**'But I was just the same as him, and I turned out fine!'**
This is a common objection, usually from the father, to the idea of his child being treated for ADHD. There is a lot we can learn from this statement. We know that ADHD is genetic, and in some respects, we should be thankful for this.

Children idolise their parents, especially little boys their fathers. I'm sure you have experienced this. If you as a parent have had ADHD, you could be the ideal life coach to help your child through it. This requires vulnerability and self-disclosure on your part. You need to share your childhood, perhaps even painful parts of it. As difficult as this might be for you, it is incredibly liberating for your child, whose self-esteem will probably have been bruised by the negative feedback associated with ADHD, and who may well be feeling very isolated as a result of the condition. Just to know that he is not alone, and someone as venerated as dad or mom had (or has) the same issues, is a weight off his shoulders. You have some important advice to give – first-hand experience – but first you have to build the platform. Self-disclosure helps to build it.

This is not unique to ADHD, as I have discovered. My children listen when I talk about myself, and especially when I reveal my weaknesses. This might require a revision of your world view; I don't apologise for this. None of us is perfect; what matters is what we do with our imperfection.

**Getting your own house in order**
If you are one of those in whom ADHD has persisted into adulthood, then you have probably noticed how frustrating certain aspects of parenting can be. It is difficult at the best of times to provide focused attention for your child,

but if you are distracted to start with, then the odds are stacked against you. Your capacity to provide routine and structure are compromised when your own time management, planning and organisational skills are poor.

Other psychiatric illnesses will also affect your parenting, and adversely affect your child's prognosis. We have already discussed the damaging effects of postnatal depression, but clinical depression or anxiety in either parent, at any stage, will interfere with effective parenting. And the same is true for any psychiatric illness. Getting proper treatment will benefit that parent and the whole family. I have often recommended that one or both parents receive treatment rather than the child who was referred to me. In many such cases, nothing else is required.

Children learn more from what we do than what we say, a phenomenon referred to as 'modelling.' They copy us. Therefore if we want our kids to be organised, focused and able to delay gratification, then we must model those qualities. If you will permit, we may be tapping into something deeper here. The French philosopher Jacques Ellul argues, in *Money and Power,* that there is a spiritual continuity between parents and their (preadolescent) children which transcends mere modelling. Our issues remain their issues – no matter how well we think we hide them – until we overcome them in ourselves. But I won't push the point.

## The lost art of apprenticeship

Now it may be that you *did* turn out fine. Congratulations, but here again there are lessons to be learnt. As we have discovered, there are a number of environmental and psychological influences which determine the prognosis in ADHD, and we need to be intentional about leveraging these for good. After all, what worked for you might well work for your child.

In years gone by, there was something honourable about following in one's father's footsteps. It was both expected and accepted for the son of a blacksmith to also become one. In the process, he was able to draw alongside his father in ways which enhanced his overall development. Today a tradesman wants his child to become a professional and works very hard to facilitate this, but in the process something else – perhaps something more important – is often sacrificed. I don't decry parents giving their children the best possible opportunities, and we should certainly not place limitations on the potential of our offspring, but a boy needs his father to help navigate the passage into manhood. I think we have forgotten much of the wisdom of apprenticeship.

## Getting organised

Most ADHD treatment guidelines recommend that non-pharmacological interventions be attempted before medication is used, especially in preschool children. Essentially, these behavioural approaches hinge on a few key concepts.

Over time, individuals with ADHD tend to acquire practical coping skills, allowing them to overcome the debilitating effects of the condition. This often happens naturally, but it can be facilitated by an intentional approach from as early on in life as possible. Again, you are the coach. In each of my kids' rooms (except the four-year-old's) is a whiteboard with a weekly planner. A brightly coloured laminated page with a marker will do the job just as well. These act as visual reminders, helping to overcome forgetfulness and absent-mindedness. It is their responsibility to check the board the evening before every school day, and prepare accordingly. It is important to encourage these and similar habits from as young as possible, and to allow the consequences to happen!

## Giving instructions

You have probably worked this one out for yourself. If you ask a child with ADHD to pack up his toys, wash his hands and come to the table, you are unlikely to get more than one out of three accomplished. This is not only due to his limited concentration, but also probably to his poor working memory; his capacity to 'hold' new auditory information in his head is impaired. Working memory forms part of the executive function network which we discussed previously. So the idea is to break up the instruction into smaller, 'bite-sized' amounts – we call it *chunking* – by giving one instruction at a time, and praising each successful component. Over time, the complexity of tasks can be gradually increased, thus exercising the 'muscle' of working memory, according to the ability of the child.

## A token economy

This is an annoying piece of jargon, which simply means a system of rewarding positive behaviour. It usually takes the form of a star chart, or for older children, a points system. The principle behind it is that a child (actually anyone) is likely to repeat the behaviours which result in a positive outcome, and desist from those which don't. It's nice when your parents are pleased with you, and when you are rewarded by the teacher. By using such strategies, we are 'catching' a child being good, as opposed to only noticing her when she annoys you in some way. It also provides an incentive for the child, and we know that children with ADHD typically require much external motivation. Once a week, say on a Saturday morning, you total up the stars or points and redeem them for a treat, a toy, a special activity, cash, airtime or whatever motivates your child.

The rewards will lose their motivating effect, of course, if they are available 'on tap' anyway, so doting grandparents need to co-operate with the system. Also, star charts will only work if they are consistently and fairly applied, and each sibling should have their own chart, even if they don't have the condition. Finally, don't be surprised if the system stops working after six months; it will need to be modified for the changing developmental stages of your child.

In case you were asking, this is *not* bribery. As an example, let's consider a child having a tantrum in a shopping centre, because you won't buy her a toy. You can allow her to make her choice and live with the consequences (no star for that day), notwithstanding your embarrassment, or you can 'bribe' her to stop by offering her an ice-cream. Positive reinforcement allows her to make the choice and aims to develop her character, by allowing her to experience the consequences of her decision, good or bad. Bribery is a form of manipulation and is actually for the parent's benefit. Of course, we can't be dependent on star charts for the rest of our lives, but this is a stage in the process of becoming a mature adult.

### Don't hide behind the diagnosis

Positive reinforcement relies on the principles of classical conditioning, made famous in animal studies. But if we leave it there, we sell ourselves short. Humans can think, reflect and make rational choices. Yes, even children! What we are implying, critically, is that children have *agency.* They can make decisions and they can exercise self-will, thus overcoming their natural inclinations. They are not at the mercy of their brain chemistry. This is very important to understand, lest we fall into the trap of 'hiding behind' the condition in a deterministic fashion, making excuses for our children, and thereby obstructing their healthy development.

**The medicalisation of naughtiness**
It seems that modern psychiatry, for all its political correctness, has medicalised bad behaviour. Hoffman's 19th century description of the 'naughty' or 'rude' child will no longer be countenanced. We have to find a diagnosis for him. This has confused and hamstrung many parents. When an ADHD child impulsively bites his sister, is it the condition or is it behavioural? So they find themselves paralysed into indecision, and default to, 'did you take your medication today?' This gives entirely the wrong message to the child, and in effect robs him of his sense of agency.

If your child is on medication, by all means administer it properly and regularly. But *after* that, it's every man for himself, so to speak. Our kids are all on the same playing field. We are preparing them for life, and the outside world won't allow such excuses. But it is harder for them, and so we use appropriate behavioural strategies to facilitate the process.

**Hectic mornings**
For parents (especially mothers) of ADHD kids, certain times of the day are particularly stressful. School mornings, for example. There is time pressure, you're not a morning person and to top it all, you have a child who daydreams, can't seem to dress independently and has no

sense of time whatsoever. What tends to happen is lots of shouting and screaming, which is not the best start to the day for you or your child.

Firstly, please turn the TV off. We have already discussed the damaging effects of the 'plug-in drug,' as it has been termed, and in the mornings it only increases the distractions on offer. The same goes for other electronic devices. Then, instead of ranting and raving, which increases everyone's stress levels and aggravates the condition, you need to offer an incentive for successfully dressing independently and getting to the breakfast table on time. It is often very helpful in the mornings to use a more concrete, tangible reminder of passing time, such as an egg-timer. This also introduces an element of fun to the morning routine and makes it less of a chore.

**Whose homework is it anyway?**
But getting homework done probably takes the cake. Your ADHD child will typically procrastinate and find excuses to avoid her work, and when she finally settles down to it, you realise she has forgotten the relevant books at school. She struggles to work without close supervision, making it difficult when there are other children to consider. The whole experience often degenerates into an unpleasant clash of wills, in which damaging words are used. In certain families, it is preferable to 'outsource' homework to a tutor or an au-pair, rather than risking the relationship between the mother (usually) and child. In many cases, if a child is on medication in the afternoons, this will facilitate the homework shift, allowing for a much smoother afternoon. But there are also important parenting principles to consider here.

I often hear mothers saying, 'I've got to get him through these exams.' Doesn't *he* need to get himself through these exams? You've already done yours. He needs to take responsibility for it and own it. As a parent you need to make peace with whatever the consequences might be, knowing that they will provide a valuable life lesson for your child. This is, after all, how they learn. If it remains your problem, the learning opportunity is lost; all he will learn is that mom uses lots of words, but in the end she will fix my mess.

## Learning from consequences
The wonderful thing about consequences is that children learn from them (they are cleverer than you think!), and their behaviour changes for the better, *provided their parents allow this to happen.* If your child doesn't study for his test, he fails; if he fails often enough, he repeats the year. It's simple cause and effect. This doesn't mean you have to sit on your hands for the whole year. As a parent, you are actively involved in setting up the consequences. For example, you might make the access to a favourite toy or activity contingent upon a minimum result (which you know he is capable of) for the weekly class test: 'You are welcome to use your X-box as soon as your grade is a "C" or better.' Then sit back, and let him decide; you don't have to shout or get scary. This set-up will require close collaboration between you and the teacher(s), but this can usually be arranged.

## Respecting the line
Allowing our children to experience the consequences of their choices calls for an awareness of interpersonal boundaries. You are free to choose, but bad choices yield unpleasant results. As parents, we need to be courageous enough and yes, respectful enough, to allow this process to happen without sabotaging it with bail-outs. This might

require a shift in the way you view discipline and relationships, but remember, our goal is to prepare our children for life, which means they need to think for themselves and generate solutions to their own problems. As Danny Silk states, in *Culture of Honor*,

> *There is a line of demarcation, and it represents where one life stops and another life starts. If we believe that we can control others or that we should, to demonstrate our great love, then there is no line...if I am to honor your life and self-control, then there must be a line where I stop and you start.*

### Reducing expressed emotion

An important byproduct of this strategy is that parental shouting and screaming is kept to a minimum. As outlined earlier, emotional volatility has a negative impact on the prognosis in ADHD. The better the quality of your relationship with your ADHD child (or any child), the better the outcome. Parental hostility interferes with this relationship. But the nature of the condition is such that it will frustrate you, unless you have a plan in place, a strategy to implement when you feel your buttons are being pushed. This requires good and regular communication between you and your spouse, and sometimes, formal parent counseling.

### Creating a culture of honour

An exciting development in the field is the emergence of several parenting programmes, designed with due regard for the established research on ADHD, such as the New Forest Parenting Programme in the UK. These are increasingly available to the general public. The advantage of the group setting is the support offered by parents in a similar predicament; there is a lot to be said for this. There are also many outstanding advocacy groups; in South Africa, ADHASA (see web address in notes) provides an excellent service to affected families.

The best parenting course I have encountered (although it is not specifically for ADHD) is that presented by Danny and Sheri Silk, entitled *Loving our kids on purpose*. Their premise is that too often, our interactions with our kids centre around *our* fear of their wrongdoing, and our need to control them. We thus resort to punishment, which disempowers our children, further eroding their self-esteem. Punishment damages the heart-to-heart connection between the parent and child, and results in shame: 'you are bad; you must pay!'

Rather, we need to create the kind of environment which protects our relationships with our kids. This environment, which they term a 'culture of honour,' is free of fear; we don't fear their wrongdoing, and they don't fear our ranting and raving. It allows us to discipline, rather than punish. Our kids' mistakes are learning opportunities; we should be thankful for them, not scared of them. Through asking effective questions rather than lecturing, and allowing them to experience consequences, we need to guide our children to generate solutions from the inside out. This is proper discipline, which *enhances* a child's self-esteem.

Such an approach has everything to do with ADHD, as it facilitates the development of agency. It says to the child: 'I believe in your ability to improve; let me help you learn from this.'

We owe our children nothing less.

# Time to get off the soapbox?

The soapbox has a place. Important children's issues need to be debated by society, and parents should be part of that process. But the debate must be informed by the facts, as far as they will take us. When emotions run high, reason is often the casualty.

As professionals, we have an obligation to present the science as honestly as possible to parents and the media, even the ambiguous and less palatable aspects, and as plainly as possible, stripped of confusing jargon. At some point, we all in turn need to climb down from the soapbox, starting with the doctor. Parents do not respond to being preached at. They require empathy and understanding; a sense of shared humanity. In the process of assessment and treatment, they need to feel heard, and we need to afford them the dignity of making an informed decision, armed with the facts.

Friends, grandparents, and other relatives, you also need to step down. I see so many parents who are too afraid to tell their family members about their child's condition or treatment. They feel isolated and alone, at a time when they most need support. Whatever your views on the matter, these parents are doing the best they can, and they need your understanding, not your condemnation.

Fellow parent, at some point you too will need to get off the soapbox, lay aside your megaphone, and simply be a parent. In many ways, this is much harder to do. But children don't learn from loudhailers; we have to find a better way. If your son or daughter has ADHD, remember you have an orchid to tend. You have been entrusted with the future. Your job is not to change the world, but to make the best decisions for your child. In so doing, you *are* helping to change the world, one child at a time.

What a fantastic opportunity!

# Further reading and acknowledgements

Books such as Malcolm Gladwell's *Outliers,* and Bill Bryson's *A Short History of Nearly Everything,* are for me, excellent examples of how to make science accessible to the layperson. Ben Goldacre's *Bad Science* is a similar achievement; I recommend it to every provider and consumer of health services (that is, everyone!).

For those looking for more information on ADHD, I heartily recommend Thomas Brown's *Attention Deficit Disorder - The Unfocused Mind in Children and Adults*; this book is particularly helpful in explaining the executive functions and their role in ADHD. I found Russell Barkley's *Your Defiant Child* to be a user-friendly guide to implementing the principles of the token economy.

The parenting course run by Danny and Sheri Silk, *Loving our kids on purpose*, is outstanding. Although Christian in its outlook, you don't have to be Christian to benefit from it. I have started to use these principles in both my home and my practice.

I am very grateful to all the children and parents who have braved my consulting room over the years. I have learnt so much from the challenging questions you have posed. I hope I have provided you with some answers.

My friends Iain, Steve, Graham, Chris, Colin, Andrew, both Gareths, Themba, James and Phiway: thank you for encouraging me all the way. All those family and friends who have helped me with proof-reading and other advice, I appreciate your time and support. Thank you Paul for your expertise with the cover.

I am grateful to Professor Lynn Holford who taught me child psychiatry, and continues to challenge me to see the wood for the trees.

My colleagues Kedi, Angie, Androula and Sonja, and my receptionists Annemien and Louise, thanks for stepping into the breach and allowing me the time off to do this.

Most importantly, I would not have been able to complete this task without the patience and support of my wife, Debby, and my children, Emma, Damian, Chloë and David.

Thank you!

# Notes

**Chapter 1:     Fidgety Philip and the history of ADHD**

1          Alexander Crichton, *An inquiry into the nature
           and origin of mental derangement:
           comprehending a concise system of the physiology
           and pathology of the human mind and a history of
           the passions and their effects.* (1798)

3          Hoffmann H, English edition: *Slovenly Peter or
           cheerful stories and funny pictures for good little
           folks.* Free ebook at:http://www.gutenberg.org

4          George Frederick Still, Some abnormal psychical
           conditions in children: the Goulstonian lectures.
           The Lancet (1902); 1: 1008-1012

5          '40% of boys with ADHD have Oppositional':
           Jensen PS, et al. Comorbidity in ADHD:
           implications for research, practice, and DSM-V.
           Journal of the American Academy of Child and
           Adolescent Psychiatry (1997); 36(8): 1065-79

5          'association between ADHD and lower IQ':
           Wood AC, et al. The relationship between ADHD
           and key cognitive phenotypes is not mediated by
           shared familial effects with IQ. Psychological
           Medicine (2011); 41(4): 861-71

## Chapter 2: 'Please test him for ADHD'

10     'qEEG':
       At least in South Africa, it has become
       fashionable to use this as a diagnostic strategy,
       despite the lack of supporting evidence.

10     Diagnostic and Statistical Manual of Mental
       Disorder, Volume IV. American Psychiatric
       Association (1994)

13     Rating scales
       http://www.neurotransmitter.net/adhdscales.html

15     'nine distinct dimensions of temperament':
       Stella Chess and Alexander Thomas, *Know Your
       Child: An Authoritative Guide For Today's
       Parents*. New York Basic Books (1987)

## Chapter 3: Orchids and dandelions

18     Family studies, twin studies and adoption studies:
       Stergiakouli E and Thapar A. Fitting the pieces
       together: current research on the genetic basis of
       attention-deficit/hyperactivity disorder (ADHD).
       Neuropsychiatric Disease and Treatment (2010);
       6: 551–560.

20     'We know this because of sophisticated imaging':
       Mahone EM et al. A Preliminary Neuroimaging
       Study of Preschool Children with ADHD. The
       Clinical Neuropsychologist (2011); 25(6): 1009-
       1028

23    'A mother's smoking or drinking in pregnancy':
      Kooij SJ et al. European consensus statement on
      diagnosis and treatment of adult ADHD: The
      European Network Adult ADHD. BMC
      Psychiatry (2010); 10: 67

24    'steer clear of it':
      In David Dobbs, *The Science of Success*,
      December 2009. www.theatlantic.com

25    'Harry Harlow':
      http://psychclassics.yorku.ca/Harlow/love.htm

26    'facilitates healthy relationships in childhood':
      Lyons-Ruth et al. Disorganized infant attachment
      classification and maternal psychosocial problems
      as predictors of hostile-aggressive behavior in the
      preschool classroom. Child Development (1993);
      64(2): 572-85

26    'longer attention spans and show more persistence
      in tasks':
      Frankel KA, Bates JE. Mother-toddler problem
      solving: antecedents in attachment, home
      behavior, and temperament. Child Development
      (1990); 61(3): 810-9

27    'support an association between insecure
      attachment and ADHD':
      Clark L et al. Attention deficit hyperactivity
      disorder is associated with attachment insecurity.
      Clinical child psychology and psychiatry (2002)

27     'Donald Winnicott':
       http://en.wikipedia.org/wiki/Donald_Winnicott

28     'one study estimating the prevalence':
       Ebstein RP et al. Dopamine D4 receptor (DRD4)
       exon III polymorphism associated with the human
       personality trait of Novelty Seeking. Nature
       Genetics (1996); 12 (1): 78-80

28     Thom Hartmann, *The Edison Gene.* Park Street
       Press (2003)

29     'orchid hypothesis':
       In David Dobbs, *The Science of Success*,
       December 2009. www.theatlantic.com

29     'In contrast, orchid children':
       Ibid

30     'more sensitive to the quality of parenting':
       Sheese BE et al. Parenting quality interacts with
       genetic variation in dopamine receptor D4 to
       influence temperament in early childhood.
       Development and Psychopathology (2007); 19(4):
       1039-46

and   Bakermans-Kranenburg MJ et al. Experimental
       evidence for differential susceptibility: dopamine
       D4 receptor polymorphism (DRD4 VNTR)
       moderates intervention effects on toddlers'
       externalizing behavior in a randomized controlled
       trial. Development and Psychopathology (2008);
       44(1): 293-300

30 'epigenetic changes':
http://www.time.com/time/magazine/article/0,917
1,1952313,00.html#ixzz226KWQ1If

31 'it's the environment stupid!':
Sonuga-Barke EJ. Journal of Child Psychology
and Psychiatry (2010); 51:2: 113-115

## Chapter 4: False positives and false negatives

33 'stimulant prescriptions in the US increased':
Zuvekas SH et al. Recent trends in stimulant
medication use among U.S. children. American
Journal of Psychiatry (2006); 163(4): 579-85

33 'cognitive enhancement':
Outram SM. The use of methylphenidate among
students: the future of enhancement? Journal of
Medical Ethics (2010); 36(4): 198-202

34 'recently published paper':
Parens E, Johnston J. Facts, values, and Attention-
Deficit Hyperactivity Disorder (ADHD): an
update on the controversies. Child and Adolescent
Psychiatry and Mental Health (2009); 3:1

34 'Great Smoky Mountain':
Angold A et al. Stimulant treatment for children: a
community perspective. Journal of the American
Academy of Child and Adolescent Psychiatry
(2000); 39(8): 975-84

34 'final common pathway':
Furman L. What is attention-deficit hyperactivity
disorder (ADHD)? Journal of Child Neurology
(2005); 20(12): 994-1002

35 'shares many symptoms with ADHD':
Zepf FD. Attention deficit-hyperactivity disorder
and early-onset bipolar disorder: two facets of one
entity? Dialogues in Clinical Neuroscience
(2009); 11(1): 63-72

36 'A learning disorder':
In the UK, the term 'learning disability' refers to
globally low IQ, or mental handicap.

36 'conductor of an orchestra':
Thomas E. Brown, Ph.D. *Attention Deficit
Disorder: The Unfocused Mind in Children and
Adults*. New Haven, CT: Yale University Press
(2005)

38 'ridiculously high rate of comorbidity':
Professor Sir Michael Rutter. Eunethydis, 2nd
International Conference, Barcelona, May 2012

39 'a biological programming effect':
Rutter M et al. Are There Biological
Programming Effects for Psychological
Development? Findings from a Study of
Romanian Adoptees. Developmental Psychology
(2004); 40(1): 81–94

40     '85% of children with RAD meet criteria for':
Minnis H et al. Discrimination between attention deficit hyperactivity disorder and reactive attachment disorder in school aged children. Research in Developmental Disabilities (2011); 32(2): 520-6

41     '50% don't receive any':
Jensen PS et al. Overlooked and underserved: "action signs" for identifying children with unmet mental health needs. Pediatrics (2011); 128(5): 970-9

42     'well-documented under-identification and under-diagnosis of ADHD in girls':
Biederman J et al. Influence of gender on attention deficit hyperactivity disorder in children referred to a psychiatric clinic. The American Journal of Psychiatry (2002); 159(1): 36-42

42     'Race and ethnicity':
Cuffe SP et al. Prevalence and correlates of ADHD symptoms in the national health interview survey. Journal of Attention Disorders (2005); 9(2): 392-401

42     'these differences were independent of':
Bailey RK, Owens DL. Overcoming challenges in the diagnosis and treatment of attention-deficit/hyperactivity disorder in African Americans. Journal of the National Medical Association (2005); 97(10 Suppl): 5S-10S

## Chapter 5:    Prevention is better than cure

44      'a study published in 2005':
        Birnbaum HG et al. Costs of attention deficit-
        hyperactivity disorder (ADHD) in the US: excess
        costs of persons with ADHD and their family
        members in 2000. Current Medical Research and
        Opinion (2005); 21(2): 195-206

45      'in her acclaimed':
        Mary Gordon, *Roots of Empathy*. The Experiment
        (2009)

46      'more than 20 hours per week of non-maternal
        care':
        Belsky J, Rovine. Nonmaternal care in the first
        year of life and security of infant—parent
        attachment. Child Development (1988); 59:
        157—167

47      'it certainly is now':
        Cheng S et al. Early television exposure and
        children's behavioral and social outcomes at age
        30 months. J Epidemiol (2010); 20 (Suppl2):
        S482-9

and     Pagani LS et al. Prospective associations between
        early childhood television exposure and academic,
        psychosocial, and physical well-being by middle
        childhood. Archives of Pediatrics and Adolescent
        Medicine (2010); 164(5): 425-31

49      'recent longitudinal study of several twin pairs':
        Wong CC et al. A longitudinal study of epigenetic

variation in twins. Epigenetics (2010); 5(6): 516-526

49    'a large, randomised study evaluating ADHD treatment in several hundred preschoolers': Kollins SH et al. Rationale, design, and methods of the Preschool ADHD Treatment Study (PATS). Journal of the American Academy of Child Adolescent Psychiatry (2006); 45(11): 1275-83

50    'Like that of Jeff Halperin and his team': Halperin JM et al. Training Executive, Attention, and Motor Skills: A Proof-of-Concept Study in Preschool Children With ADHD. Journal of Attention Disorders (2012) Mar 5 [Epub ahead of print]

50    'proven benefits to the developing brain': Summarised in: Halperin JM, Healey DM. The influences of environmental enrichment, cognitive enhancement, and physical exercise on brain development: can we alter the developmental trajectory of ADHD? Neuroscience and Biobehavioral Reviews (2011); 35(3): 621-34

## Chapter 6:    Dietary strategies for ADHD

53    'documented association between ADHD and obesity': Cortese S et al. Obesity and ADHD: Clinical and Neurobiological Implications. Current Topics in Behavioural Neurosciences (2012); 9: 199-218

54    'Figure 3':
       The Muller-Lyer Illusion

55    'Nobel prizewinning researcher and writer':
       Daniel Kahnemann, *Thinking, fast and slow*.
       Penguin Books (2011)

58    'This has been well documented':
       Ben Goldacre, *Bad Science.* Fourth Estate
       London (2009)

59    'majority did not show significant benefits':
       Nigg JT et al. Meta-analysis of attention-
       deficit/hyperactivity disorder or attention-
       deficit/hyperactivity disorder symptoms,
       restriction diet, and synthetic food color additives.
       Journal of the American Academy of Child and
       Adolescent Psychiatry (2012); 51(1): 86-97

59    'randomised, placebo-controlled trial of 100
       ADHD kids':
       Pelsser LM et al. Effects of a restricted
       elimination diet on the behaviour of children with
       attention-deficit hyperactivity disorder (INCA
       study): a randomised controlled trial. The Lancet
       (2011); 377(9764): 494 - 503

60    'A recently published meta-analysis':
       Bloch MH, Qawasmi A. Omega-3 fatty acid
       supplementation for the treatment of children with
       attention-deficit/hyperactivity disorder
       symptomatology: systematic review and meta-
       analysis. Journal of the American Academy of
       Child and Adolescent Psychiatry (2011); 50(10):

991-1000

## Chapter 7    What's the fuss about medication?

64    'laments the current state of medical journalism':
      Ben Goldacre, *Bad Science*.  Fourth Estate
      London (2009)

66    'numerous well-designed':
      Ghuman JK et al. Review: methylphenidate and
      atomoxetine have similar efficacy and
      acceptability in children and adolescents with
      ADHD. Evidence Based Mental Health (2012);
      15(3): 74

68    'overall, the average reduction in height gain':
      Vitiello B. Understanding the risk of using
      medications for attention deficit hyperactivity
      disorder with respect to physical growth and
      cardiovascular function. Child and Adolescent
      Psychiatric Clinics of North America (2008);
      17(2): 459-74, xi.

68    'During the period January 1992 to February':
      Ibid

69    'Kiddie Cocaine: Behavior Drug Ritalin Abused
      by Children':
      Reported by CBS news, February 11, 2009.
      http://www.cbsnews.com/2100-204_162-
      327150.html

69    'overwhelming message from the scientific

literature':
Harty SC et al. The Impact of Conduct Disorder
and Stimulant Medication on Later Substance Use
in an Ethnically Diverse Sample of Individuals
with Attention-Deficit/Hyperactivity Disorder in
Childhood. Journal of Child and Adolescent
Psychopharmacology (2011); 21(4): 331–339

70    'stimulant treatment into adolescence is actually
      protective':
      Wilens et al. Effect of prior stimulant treatment
      for attention-deficit/hyperactivity disorder on
      subsequent risk for cigarette smoking and alcohol
      and drug use disorders in adolescents. Archives of
      Pediatrics and Adolescent Medicine (2008);
      162(10): 916-21

71    'a majority are approached to sell, trade':
      Sepúlveda DR et al. Misuse of prescribed
      stimulant medication for ADHD and associated
      patterns of substance use: preliminary analysis
      among college students. Journal of Pharmacy
      Practice (2011); 24(6): 551-60

71    'no script is required':
      At the time of writing, melatonin is available over
      the counter in South Africa, although there are
      moves afoot to change its scheduling.

73    'no completed suicides were reported':
      European guidelines group. European guidelines
      on managing adverse effects of medication for
      ADHD. European Child and Adolescent
      Psychiatry (2011); 20(1): 17–37

73    'ADHD is itself associated with an increased risk of suicidality':
Lahey B et al. Very early predictors of Adolescent Depression and Suicide Attempts in Children with Attention-Deficit/Hyperactivity Disorder.
Archives of General Psychiatry (2010); 67(10): 1044-1051

77    'an educational study':
Malcolm Gladwell, *Outliers: The Story of Success*. Penguin Books (2008)

79    'persists into adulthood in at least 60% of cases':
Kooij SJ et al. European consensus statement on diagnosis and treatment of adult ADHD: The European Network Adult ADHD. BMC Psychiatry (2010); 10: 67

## Chapter 8    Parenting a child with ADHD

83    'tapping into something deeper here':
Jacques Ellul, *Money and Power*. Inter-Varsity Press (1984)

88    'plug-in drug':
Marie Winn, *The Plug-in Drug*. New York: Penguin Books (1977)

90    Danny Silk, *Culture of Honor: sustaining a supernatural environment*. Destiny Image publishers (2009)

90   'New Forest Parenting Programme':
     http://education.gov.uk/commissioning-
     toolkit/Programme/Detail/41

91   'ADHASA':
     http://www.adhdsupport.co.za/

91   'Loving our kids on purpose':
     Danny Silk, *Loving our kids on purpose*. Destiny
     Image Publishers (2008)

# About the author

Brendan Belsham is a child and adolescent psychiatrist in private practice in Johannesburg. He trained at the University of the Witwatersrand, winning awards for psychiatry as an undergraduate and postgraduate student.

He has appeared on television, spoken on radio and written for magazines. His special interests include ADHD, early parenting, attachment, autism and anxiety disorders.

He is married with four children.

Made in the USA
Charleston, SC
28 September 2012